DANA CARPENDER'S

NEW CARB & CALORIE COUNTER

**EXPANDED
REVISED
UPDATED
FOURTH EDITION**

Text © 2010 Dana Carpender

First published in the USA in 2009 by
Fair Winds Press, a member of
Quayside Publishing Group
100 Cummings Center
Suite 406-L
Beverly, MA 01915-6101
www.fairwindspress.com

14 13 12 11 10   1 2 3 4 5

ISBN-13: 978-1-59233-429-2
ISBN-10: 1-59233-429-6

Library of Congress Cataloging-in-Publication Data available

Edited by Erika Bruce
Cover design by BradhamDesign.com
Original book design by Leslie Haimes and tabula rasa
Book Design by Yee Design

Printed and bound in Canada

*The information in this book is for educational purposes only. It is not
intended to replace the advice of a physician or medical practitioner. Please
see your health care provider before beginning any new health program.*

Note: The data is accurate at the time of publication. However, food
manufacturers may change their ingredients at any time without notice.

DANA CARPENDER'S

NEW CARB & CALORIE COUNTER

EXPANDED
REVISED
UPDATED
FOURTH EDITION

Your
Complete Guide to
TOTAL CARBS
NET CARBS
CALORIES
and More

DANA CARPENDER
Author of the best-selling *500 Low-Carb Recipes*

FAIR WINDS
PRESS
BEVERLY, MASSACHUSETTS

Contents

Introduction

Hello, low-carb dieter! Whether you're new to the low-carb lifestyle, or have been doing this for a while, I hope you'll find this book a useful tool to achieving weight loss, abundant energy, and robust good health.

I've written a *lot* of words about the low-carbohydrate lifestyle in the past few years, and I won't try to repeat them all here. But I would like to offer the condensed version, as it were—what I feel are the most vital tips for low-carb success.

Know The Basics

- First, and perhaps most important, get clear on this: Whatever you do to lose weight is what you must do for *the rest of your life* to keep it off. And if carbs are a problem for you now, they will continue to be a health problem for you until the day you die. Always remind yourself that *there is no finish line.*

- Because you're in this for life, don't focus on losing your weight as quickly as possible. Instead, work on making low-carbing the enjoyable lifestyle it can be, while still achieving your goals. In particular, do *not* decide that if low-carb is good, then no carb must be better, and cut out everything but eggs, meat, and cheese. You can't eat that way forever, and you know it. You need to incorporate the widest variety of low-carb foods you can, to add flavor and interest, not to mention vitamins, minerals, and fiber.

- It's important to know about what are called "impact carbs," "useable carbs," "net carbs," or "effective carbs." These terms all refer to the grams of carbohydrate that you can actually digest and absorb. What carbohydrates can't you digest or absorb? Fiber! The carbohydrate chains that make up dietary fibers are just too big for the human gut to digest and absorb, which is why we can't live on grass like cows do. Accordingly, you can subtract the grams of fiber from the total grams of carbohydrate to get the number of grams of carbohydrate you actually need to worry about. In this book, we call this number "net carbs." This approach dramatically increases the amount of vegetables, fruits, nuts, seeds, and other plant foods you can eat.

- It is my experience that a low-carbohydrate diet is a superb way to overcome genuine obesity and the health problems that come with it—but it's not particularly useful for achieving that fashionably malnourished look. If you're a size 4 trying to become a size 0, I probably can't help you, and furthermore, I don't want to! It's about *health*, not about making yourself vanish!

- If you're new to low-carbing, be aware that the first week can be rough. If, like most people, you've been giving your body a little carbohydrate every few hours, your body is used to running on sugar, and probably hasn't been making much of the enzymes you need to burn fat for fuel. If you burn through your body's stores of sugar before your fat-burning enzyme levels increase, you may "bonk"—feel terribly tired and wrung-out for a day or two. Not everyone goes through this (I didn't) but if it happens to you, know that for most people it lasts no more than few days. When it's over, you'll be burning fat for fuel, and have more energy than you ever imagined, because you're carrying your supply with you!

- If along with feeling tired, you feel kind of achy, weak, or crampy, then potassium loss—called "hypokalemia"—is likely to be your problem. And if this happens to you, get more potassium *right away*. Your heart needs potassium to run properly! *Don't mess around*. The best low-carb source of potassium is avocados; one California avocado (the black-skinned ones) has 2.5 grams of net carbs and 660 milligrams of potassium. Green leafy vegetables are also a good low-carb source of potassium, as is fresh pork, fresh fish, cantaloupe, and almonds. Indeed, it's best to include these things in your diet from day one.

    You can also take potassium tablets, if you like, but be aware that the doses tend to be low, at just 99 milligrams per tablet, when you need 2000 to 3000 milligrams of potassium per day. Another way to supplement is to use Morton's Lite Salt, which combines the usual sodium-based salt with potassium-based salt. (CAUTION: If you are on blood pressure medication of any kind, check with your pharmacist or doctor before taking potassium supplements. Some blood pressure medications work by making your body hang on to potassium, and that makes it possible to get too much, which is as dangerous as too little.)

    Note that potassium imbalance is a temporary problem, caused by your body's shifting over from a high-carb diet, which makes you throw off potassium and retain water, to a low-carb diet, which makes you dump all that excess water before your body stops throwing off the potassium. Just eat your good potassium sources, and your body will sort it all out in a week or two.

Tips for Finding YOUR Low-Carb Lifestyle

- There are many approaches to controlling carbohydrates in your diet. If all you've heard about is Atkins and/or The South Beach Diet, and you've been unhappy or uncomfortable on these diets, don't give up—do some research, and find the approach that works for your body and your life. In my book *How I Gave Up My Low Fat Diet and Lost 40 Pounds*, I outline more than a half a dozen different approaches to controlling your carbohydrate intake, and therefore your insulin levels. No need for a one-size-fits-all diet.

- Pay attention to your body to learn your "critical carbohydrate level"—the number of grams per day of carbohydrate you must stay below in order to lose weight. For most people this will be between 15 and 60 grams per day. Only time and attention will tell you your critical carbohydrate level.

- You can get an idea of where your critical carbohydrate level is likely to be by checking how many of the signs of carbohydrate intolerance you have. Here's a list of indicators, things that have been linked to carb intolerance. How many apply to you?

    ___ I have had a weight problem since I was young.

    ___ I have bad energy slumps, especially in the late afternoon.

    ___ I get tired and/or shaky when I get hungry.

__ I'm depressed and irritable for no reason.

__ I binge badly or frequently on carbohydrate foods.

__ I carry most of my weight on my abdomen.

__ I have high blood pressure.

__ I have high triglycerides.

__ I have high cholesterol.

__ I have adult onset diabetes.

__ I have heart disease.

__ I have had a female cancer (breast, cervical, ovarian, uterine).

__ I have had a stroke.

__ I am an alcoholic.

__ I have polycystic ovarian syndrome, or the symptoms of it.

__ Obesity runs in my family.

__ High blood pressure runs in my family.

__ High triglycerides run in my family.

__ High cholesterol runs in my family.

__ Adult onset diabetes runs in my family.

__ Heart disease runs in my family.

__ Female cancers run in my family (breast, cervical, ovarian, uterine).

__ Stroke runs in my family.

__ Alcoholism runs in my family.

__ Polycystic ovarian syndrome runs in my family.

If your answer was "yes" to more than two or three of these, you're likely to be pretty carbohydrate intolerant. The more yes answers, the more intolerant you're likely to be. And the more people in your family have these problems, the more intolerant you're likely to be. Keep this in mind when choosing an approach.

- If you have any of the health issues listed above as signs of carbohydrate intolerance, it is *imperative* that you be under a doctor's supervision during at least the first few months of going low-carb. Blood pressure can come down so quickly that if your medication isn't adjusted, you'll get dizzy. Your customary dosage of diabetes medication may suddenly be enough to drop your blood sugar uncomfortably low. If you have trouble with high cholesterol and triglycerides, you need a baseline to work from or you won't know if you've gotten better or worse. Be smart. If your doctor won't cooperate, find one that will, but don't fly blind.

- Most people see an across-the-board improvement in their coronary risk factors—cholesterol, triglycerides, and HDL/LDL ratio—on a low-carb diet, even when eating red meat and high-fat dairy foods. However, a minority will see a decrease in triglycerides and an increase in HDL (the "good" cholesterol), which is good, but also see a jump in their LDL (the "bad" cholesterol), which is not so good. If this happens to you, weight your low-carb diet in favor of fish, poultry, and pork Also, use lean cuts when eating beef or lamb, and choose olive oil, nuts, and avocados—good sources of monounsaturated fat—over butter, sour cream, and cheese.

Tricks to Staying Happy

- In the pursuit of low-carb happiness, especially in the early stages, sit down and brainstorm a list of all of your favorite low-carb foods. What foods do you really love that you've been denying yourself because they were high-fat and high-calorie? Lobster with butter? Macadamia nuts? Deviled eggs? Brie? Really give this list some thought. Then buy or cook this stuff, and eat it! It's a great way to stave off feelings of deprivation.

- Buy at least one low-carb cookbook, such as my best-selling book *500 Low-Carb Recipes*. People tell me they like it because it doesn't call for a lot of weird ingredients, and has a lot of simple recipes that their families like. But there are plenty of other low-carb cookbooks on the market, many of them quite good. The point is, start exploring your kitchen options, instead of letting yourself get locked into fried eggs for breakfast, a bunless burger for lunch, and a plain steak for dinner.

- Make a list of ways to reward yourself that don't involve food. A massage, an hour in a hot bath with a good book, a manicure and pedicure, a phone call to an old friend you haven't talked to in forever—whatever you can think of that will make you feel rewarded, but won't make you fat, sick, and tired. When you've had a hard week, or reached a personal goal, give yourself one of these rewards, instead of carb-filled treat that will only hurt you in the long run.

- When you've lost your first ten or fifteen pounds, buy yourself something wonderful and new to wear—it's a terrific incentive.

It's not a bad idea to do this every time you drop another size, if you can afford it, rather than waiting until you've reached your goal weight to buy new clothes. New clothes celebrate and show off your success, and keep you on track.

Know Your Labels

- Read the labels on *everything* you put in your mouth. Most people do far more research before buying a car or a DVD player than they do on what they put into their own bodies. "You are what you eat" is literally true. All your body has to make itself from is what you put in your mouth. If you give your body junk, you'll be made out of junk, and you'll feel and look like it. Read the labels, even on things you've looked up in this book or have purchased before, as formulas often change.

- Having read the labels, choose the products with the lowest carb counts. You can shave thousands of grams off of your yearly intake this way. For example, I have seen ham with 1 gram of carbohydrate per serving, and I have seen ham with 6 grams of carbohydrate per serving. That's a 600% difference!

- There is no such thing as good sugar! Obviously, sugar, brown sugar, and corn syrup are all bad for you. However, so are the "natural" and "healthy" alternatives like honey, concentrated fruit juice, Sucanat, dried sugar cane juice, malt syrup, rice syrup, turbinado, fructose, dextrose, maltose, or anything else ending in "ose." All of it is sugar, and all of it will cause an insulin release.

- Many alcoholic beverages quote low-carb counts on the labels, and hard liquor, technically speaking, has none. However, alcohol, no matter how low-carb, will slow your metabolism dramatically—you'll stop burning fat until your body has metabolized all of the alcohol. That doesn't mean that you can never have a light beer or a glass of dry wine, but it does mean that alcohol is always a major luxury on any kind of weight loss diet. You have been warned.

- Keep a close eye on the portion sizes listed on labels. Often what you assume is one serving is really two or three—which means you'll get two or three times as much carbohydrate as you bargained for.

- It's important to know that just because a food says it has "0 grams of carbohydrate" per serving, doesn't mean that it's 100% carbohydrate free. How can this be? Again, it has to do with portion size. The US federal government standards allow labels to say "0 grams" if the food contains 0.4 grams or less per serving, and "<1 gram" (less than 1 gram) if the food contains 0.9 grams or less per serving. Yet we often use these foods in larger quantities, and the grams add up.

  A perfect example: A reader of mine wanted to know where the carbs in my Margarita Mix (*500 Low-Carb Recipes*) came from—after all, lime juice, lemon juice, and Splenda all had zero grams of carbohydrate. Only they don't; they all have carbs! They only look like they're carb-free because the serving sizes used on the labels are so small. When in doubt count 0.5 grams per serving for foods that say 0 grams on the label, and 1 gram for foods that say <1 gram on the label.

- Be aware that there have been more than a few cases of mislabeled "low-carb" products that have turned out to be a lot higher in carbohydrate than the labels let on. If you add a new product to your diet and you bump up a pound or two, or find yourself hungry and craving, take a closer look—and remember that if it seems too good to be true, it just might be.

- This warning also applies to imported food products. Labeling laws vary from country to country, and much of the world does not include fiber counts in the total carb count on nutrition labels—so if you subtract the fiber count from the total carb count, you'll get an inaccurately low total, and eat more carbohydrate than you meant to. Buyer beware.

The Most Important Low-Carb Diet Element: Common Sense

- The notion that you can eat unlimited quantities of food so long as you keep the carb count very low has been oversold. It does appear to be true that you can eat *more* calories on a low-carb diet than you could on a carb-containing diet and still lose weight, but that doesn't mean you can eat 10,000 calories a day and still lose weight. So don't eat for entertainment! Eat when you're hungry, eat enough to feel satisfied, then quit until you're physically hungry again. It's a shame that we even need to be told this, it's so basic, but our society has developed a bad habit of eating for the fun of it, regardless of hunger. Cut it out!

- Americans have been programmed to eat for entertainment—snacking for long periods of time on nutritionally empty junk food, whether they're hungry or not. Low-carb foods are *filling*, and tend to be calorie-dense, and as a result, there are few low-carb foods that you can nosh on for hours without making yourself ill. If you really must have something to nibble on for hours and hours, your best bet is very low-carb vegetables, like celery and cucumber sticks. Pumpkin and sunflower seeds *in the shell* are another good choice, because having to open each individual shell slows down your consumption dramatically, and keeps your hands busy to boot. Better yet, find something else to do for entertainment!

- The heart and soul of your nutritional program, for the rest of your life, should be meat, fish, poultry, eggs and cheese, healthy fats, low-carbohydrate vegetables, low-sugar fruits, and nuts and seeds. You know—*food*. A sugar-free candy bar or brownie or a bag of low-carb chips is *never* a substitute for a chicken Caesar salad for lunch.

A Note on Low Carbohydrate/Sugar Free Specialty Products

- Roughly half of low-carbohydrate dieters find that diet soda and diet fruit-flavored beverages like Crystal Light will slow or stop their weight loss. Many also find that these beverages act as a "trigger"—something that sets off their carb cravings. Why this happens is controversial; some theorize that aspartame is to blame, while others feel that citric acid, widely used as a flavoring in these products, interferes with ketosis. Still others claim that just the taste of sweetness can cause an insulin release, whether there's any sugar involved or not. But the actual reason is unimportant—just know that if you're struggling, one of the first places to look is your diet soda consumption.

- Do not make low-carb specialty products a major part of your diet. Low-carb breads, pastas, candy, cookies, protein bars, and so on, are flooding onto the market, and they do provide a nice variety. However, most of these products are not as nutritious, healthful, or filling as real food. (Almost all of them have more carbohydrate in them than a hard-boiled egg or a chicken wing.) Furthermore, they're all extremely expensive! So stop trying to make your low-carb diet look like your old high-carb diet—that's the diet that got you in trouble in the first place, remember?

- When you hit a plateau, lose the treats. The sugar-free chocolate bars, the low-carb baked goods, and so on should be the first things to axe if you're not losing.

- Regarding those sugar-free chocolate bars, protein bars, jelly beans, brownies, etc, etc, etc: Just about all of them are sweetened with polyols, sometimes called sugar alcohols. These are carbohydrates, but they're carbohydrates that are slowly and incompletely absorbed, at most. Because of this, most low-carbers and all low-carb specialty food labels subtract out polyols from the total carb count, just like fiber. Polyol sweetened treats are easier on your body than the sugar sweetened kind, but it's optimistic to assume that none of that carbohydrate is absorbed. When low-carb sweets say you can subtract out *all* of the sugar alcohols from the carb count, take that with a grain of salt.

Also be aware that polyols/sugar alcohols often cause gas and/or diarrhea. Be very careful with your portions—I rarely eat more than a half of a 1.5-ounce chocolate bar in a day. Don't eat sugar-free sweets at all before a big job interview, an important presentation, a hot date, or getting on a plane, or you may well be sorry.

- Don't be fooled by the fact that many alcoholic drinks have a low carb count. Alcohol in any form will slow fat-burning dramatically. That doesn't mean you can't drink at all, but just realize that alcohol is *always* a major luxury on a weight loss, and gauge your intake accordingly.

Tips for Success When You're Away From Home

- Make the best choice possible given any particular circumstance. What do I mean? If you're at work, and the vending machine has cookies, crackers, chips, candy, and peanuts, then the peanuts are the best choice, even though they're relatively high-carb for a nut (because, of course, they're really a legume!). When you're genuinely hungry, and faced with foods which are not ideal for the diet, choose the food that will cause the least damage to your diet. Don't be afraid to pick off breading, eat only the cheese and toppings off the pizza, ask for an extra salad in place of the potato, and so on.

- Always remember that restaurants are in a service industry. Ask questions about ingredients if you're not certain what's in a dish. Do not hesitate to ask for low-carb substitutions, within reason—steamed vegetables in place of the potato, a bed of lettuce instead of rice, or whatever will make your meal low-carb, delicious, and satisfying. If the waiter or the kitchen gives you grief, go spend your money elsewhere. And if they're nice about it—as most restaurants are—be effusive with your praise, and tip well!

- Be polite but firm with people who want you to cheat on your diet. If you're embarrassed about asking for food exactly the way you want it at a restaurant, or about letting your friends know about your food restrictions before a dinner party, let me ask you this: If you had a deadly allergy, one that would cause you to go into anaphylactic shock at the mere *taste* of the wrong food, would you hesitate to bring it up to a waiter or a friend? Of course not, and no one would expect you to.

  Well, the truth is, more people die of the effects of carbohydrate intolerance-related diseases—heart disease, stroke, diabetes, cancer—than anything else. *Your carbohydrate intolerance is just as deadly as the severest allergy.* It just takes longer, that's all. Don't be ashamed to take care of yourself.

  I find that it's often easier to say, "I'm afraid I can't have that" than to say, "Oh, no thanks, I'm on a diet." People are far less likely to argue if you make it sound medical—which it is!

- When you're traveling, pack some "friendly" food in your purse or carry-on bag. Carry individually wrapped string cheese, a protein bar or two, some Just-The-Cheese Chips, a packet or two of nuts or seeds, or anything else that will get you through if the interval between meals gets stretched out unbearably.

10 Great Snacks for 5 grams of Net Carbs Or Less!

Two tablespoons hummus and 1 tablespoon chopped olives mixed together, served on top of ½ cup cucumber slices: 7 grams carbs, 2 grams fiber, 5 grams net carbs, 3 grams protein, 4 grams fat, 70 calories.

One slice turkey and 1 slice cheddar (1 oz), spread with 1 teaspoon mustard, and rolled up in 1 leaf butter lettuce: 2 grams carbs, 1 gram fiber, 1 gram net carbs, 11 grams protein, 10 grams fat, 140 calories.

Hard-boiled egg, one: <1 gram carbs, 0 grams fiber, <1 gram net carbs, 6 grams protein, 5 grams fat, 78 calories.
Turning that egg into a deviled egg with a little mayo and mustard will add less than 1 gram of carbohydrate!

Frozen hot wings, 3 pieces: 1 gram carbs, 0 grams fiber, 1 gram net carbs, 21 grams protein, 15 grams fat, 230 calories.
* Avoid barbecue wings—barbecue sauce is sugary.

Roasted almonds, ⅓ cup: 9 grams carb, 5 grams fiber, 4 grams net carb, 10 grams protein, 24 grams fat, 275 calories.

One ounce blue cheese and 1 ounce cream cheese, and stuffed into 1 large celery rib: 4 grams carbs, 1 gram fiber, 3 grams net carbs, 8 grams protein, 18 grams fat, 207 calories.

Pumpkin seeds, 1 ounce: **4 grams carbs**, 1 gram fiber, 3 grams net carbs, 9 grams protein, 12 grams fat, 150 calories.
Pumpkorn brand comes in great flavors!

Deluxe mixed nuts (w/o peanuts), 1 ounce: 6 grams carbs, 1 gram fiber, 5 grams net carb, 4 grams protein, 16 grams fat, 174 calories.

String cheese, 1-ounce stick: 1 gram carbs, 0 grams fiber, 1 gram net carbs, 18 grams protein, 6 grams fat, 80 calories.

Hot dog (no bun of course!), Oscar Mayer brand: 1 gram carbs, 0 grams fiber, 1 gram net carbs, 5 grams protein, 14 grams fat, 147 calories.

10 Treats for 10 Grams or Less

Sugar-free ice pop, 1 stick: 3 grams carbs, 0 grams fiber, 3 grams net carbs, 0 grams protein, 0 grams fat, 12 calories.

Six large strawberries with ½ cup whipped cream (no sugar): 10 grams carbs, 2 grams fiber, 8 grams net carbs, 2 grams protein, 23 grams fat, 242 calories.

One serving sugar-free instant pudding made with half heavy cream, half water: 2 grams carbs, 0 grams fiber, 2 grams net carbs, 1 gram protein, 205 calories.

One-eighth medium cantaloupe, sprinkled with 1 tablespoon lime juice and 1 packet Splenda: 8 grams carbs, 1 gram fiber, 7 grams net carbs, <1 gram protein, <1 gram fat, 30 calories.

Sugar-free fudge pop, 1 stick: 10 grams carbs, 2 grams fiber, 8 grams net carbs, 1 gram protein, 1 gram fat, 40 calories.

Popcorn, 2 cups, air popped: 12 grams carbs, 2 grams fiber, 10 grams net carbs, 2 grams protein, <1 gram fat, 62 calories.

Plain lowfat yogurt (½ cup) mixed with 1 packet Splenda and ½ teaspoon vanilla extract, topped with 1 tablespoon flaxseed and 1 tablespoon chopped, toasted pecans: 13 grams carbs, 3 grams fiber, 10 grams net carbs, 8 grams protein, 11 grams fat, 180 calories.

Coffee granita (1 cup strongly brewed coffee sweetened with 1 packet Splenda, frozen and then shaved with a fork), topped with 2 tablespoons whipped cream: 1 gram carbs, 0 gram fiber, 1 gram net carbs, <1 gram protein, 6 grams fat, 60 calories.

Five Reese's miniature sugar-free peanut butter cups: 23 grams carbs, 1 gram fiber, 19 grams polyols, 3 grams net carbs, 2 grams protein, 170 calories.

Seventeen Jelly Belly sugar-free jelly beans: 18 grams carbs, 4 grams fiber, 12 grams polyols, 2 grams net carbs, 0 grams protein, 0 grams fat, 40 calories.
This is half of what the Jelly Belly company lists as a serving size, but since these are so polyol-rich, I fear that eating 35 jelly beans would cause gastric upset in many people!

Lowest-Carb Fast Food Meals

For a more complete list of fast food that will work for a low-carb diet, see page 155—these are just the very lowest-carb choices at each of the biggest chains.

A&W

Corn dog nuggets, 5 pieces: 20 grams carbss, 1 gram fiber, 19 grams net carbss, 5 grams protein, 8 grams fat, 180 calories.

Arby's

Chopped Farmhouse Grilled Chicken Salad with Buttermilk Ranch Dressing: 12 grams carbs, 3 grams fiber, 9 grams net carbs, 22 grams protein, 36 grams fat, 480 calories.

Au Bon Pain

Chef's salad with light ranch dressing: 10 grams carbs, 3 grams fiber, 7 grams net carbs, 26 grams protein, 26 grams fat, 370 calories.

Gazpacho, 12 ounce portion: 11 grams carbs, 3 grams fiber, 8 grams net carbs, 2 grams protein, 5 grams fat, 90 calories.

Blimpie

Chicken Caesar salad with creamy Caesar dressing: 8 grams carbs, 3 grams fiber, 5 grams net carbs, 26 grams protein, 29 grams fat, 400 calories.

Boston Market

Beef Brisket Meal: 1 gram carbs, 0 grams fiber, 1 gram net carbs, 26 grams protein, 20 grams fat, 280 calories.

Bruegger's
Spinach & lentil soup, 1 cup: 16 grams carbs, 7 grams fiber, 9 grams net carbs, 7 grams protein, 4 grams fat, 110 calories.

Burger King
Tendergrill Chicken Garden Salad, with Ken's Light Italian dressing (dressing included): 13 grams carbs, 3 grams fiber, 10 grams net carbs, 29 grams protein, 18 grams fat, 330 calories.

Carl's Jr.
The Low Carbs Six Dollar Burger: 7 grams carbs, 1 gram fiber, 6 grams net carbs, 38 grams protein, 43 grams fat, 570 calories.

Checkers
All-beef hot dog: 23 grams carbs, 2 grams fiber, 21 grams net carbs, 11 grams protein, 17 grams fat, 280 calories.

Church's Chicken
Original chicken breast with a side of collard greens: 8 grams carbs, 3 grams fiber, 5 grams net carbs, 24 grams protein, 11 grams fat, 225 calories.

Dairy Queen
Grilled Chicken Wrap: 9 grams carbs, 1 gram fiber, 8 grams net carbs, 12 grams protein, 12 grams fat, 200 calories.
Fudge Bar, no sugar added: 13 grams carbs, 6 grams fiber, 7 grams net carbs, 4 grams protein, 0 grams fat, 50 calories.

Denny's
Top Sirloin Steak & Eggs: 1 gram carbs, 0 grams fiber, 1 gram net carbs, 54 grams protein, 21 grams fat, 420 calories.

Einstein Bros Bagels
Cup of chicken noodle soup: 14 grams carbs, 1 gram fiber, 13 grams net carbs, 5 grams protein, 4 grams fat, 120 calories.
Caesar salad: 18 grams carbs, 4 grams fiber, 14 grams net carbs, 18 grams protein, 63 grams fat, 690 calories.

El Pollo Loco
Skinless chicken breast meal: 12 grams carbs, 4 grams fiber, 8 grams net carbs, 39 grams protein, 8 grams fat, 280 calories.

Fatburger
Fatburger, no bun: 10 grams carbs, 2 grams fiber, 8 grams net carbs, 28 grams protein, 29 grams fat, 410 calories.

Friendly's
Tri-tip steak with 2 eggs, sunny-side up: 1 gram carbs, 0 grams fiber, 1 gram net carbs, 57 grams protein, 33 grams fat, 530 calories.

Hardee's
⅓ lb. Low-Carb Thickburger: 5 grams carbs, 2 grams fiber, 3 grams net carbs, 30 grams protein, 32 grams fat, 420 calories.

In-N-Out Burger
Cheeseburger with onion, "Protein" style (lettuce, no bun): 11 grams carbs, 3 grams fiber, 8 grams net carbs, 18 grams protein, 25 grams fat, 330 calories.

Jack in the Box
Grilled Chicken Breast Strips, 4 pieces: 3 grams carbs, 0 grams fiber, 3 grams net carbs, 37 grams protein, 19 grams fat, 180 calories.

Jason's Deli
Bowl of Texas chili: 20 grams carbs, 6 grams fiber, 14 grams net carbs, 35 grams protein, 20 grams fat, 400 calories.

KFC
Grilled Chicken Breast and a House Side Salad with Heinz Buttermilk Ranch Dressing (dressing included): 3 grams carbs, 1 gram fiber, 2 grams net carbs, 36 grams protein, 21 grams fat, 355 calories.

Long John Silver's
Shrimp Scampi: 1 gram carbs, 0 grams fiber, 1 gram net carbs, 16 grams protein, 5 grams fat, 110 calories.

McDonald's
Premium Bacon Ranch Salad w/ Grilled Chicken and Newman's Own Low Fat Balsamic Vinaigrette (dressing included): 16 grams carbs, 3 grams fiber, 13 grams net carbs, 33 grams protein, 12 grams fat, 300 calories.

Panda Express

Broccoli Chicken (without rice): 11 grams carbs, 3 grams fiber, 8 grams net carbs, 13 grams protein, 9 grams fat, 180 calories.

Panera Bread

Chopped chicken Cobb salad with fat-free, reduced sugar, poppyseed dressing (dressing included): 13 grams carbs, 4 grams fiber, 9 grams net carbs, 36 grams protein, 35 grams fat, 505 calories.

Pizza Hut

Baked Hot Wings, 4 pieces: 2 grams carbs, 0 grams fiber, 2 grams net carbs, 22 grams protein, 14 grams fat, 240 calories.

Baked Mild Wings, 4 pieces: 2 grams carbs, 0 grams fiber, 2 grams net carbs, 22 grams protein, 14 grams fat, 220 calories.

Popeyes Louisiana Kitchen

Chicken étouffée: 6 grams carbs, 2 grams fiber, 4 grams net carbs, 12 grams protein, 10 grams fat, 160 calories.

Sonic

Grilled chicken salad with Hidden Valley original ranch dressing (dressing included): 14 grams carbs, 3 grams fiber, 11 grams net carbs, 30 grams protein, 30 grams fat, 440 calories.

Steak-N-Shake

Chicken Chef Salad: 11 grams carbs, 3 grams fiber, 7 grams net carbs, 36 grams protein, 472 calories.

Subway
Oven Roasted Chicken Breast with Ranch Dressing (dressing included): 13 grams carbs, 4 grams fiber, 9 grams net carbs, 21 grams protein, 33 grams fat, 420 calories.

Taco Bell
Crunchy Taco: 12 grams carbs, 3 grams fiber, 9 grams net carbs, 8 grams protein, 10 grams fat, 170 calories.

Tim Horton's
Bowl of hearty vegetable soup: 14 grams carbs, 3 grams fiber, 11 grams net carbs, 4 gram protein, 0 grams fat, 70 calories.

Togo's
Farmer's Market salad with spicy pepitas dressing (dressing included): 23 grams carbs, 5 grams fiber, 18 grams net carbs, 10 grams protein, 41 grams fat, 500 calories.

Wendy's
Chicken Caesar Salad with Supreme Caesar dressing (dressing included): 9 grams carbs, 3 grams fiber, 6 grams net carbs, 29 grams protein, 17 grams fat, 300 calories.

Whataburger
Taquito with bacon, egg, and cheese: 27 grams carbs, 3 grams fiber, 24 grams net carbs, 19 grams protein, 24 grams fat, 420 calories.

How to Use This Book

This book is designed to help you count calories, carbohydrates, and nutrients accurately, quickly, and easily. Alphabetical listings make locating your foods simple. To improve clarity and speed in locating food choices, this book is divided into three sections:

Beverages
Foods
Fast Food Restaurants

Abbreviation Key

appx	approximately
as prep	prepared as instructed on package, usual method
avg	average size
bev	beverage
cal	calorie
dia	diameter
fl oz	fluid ounce
g	gram(s)
"	inch(es)
Lb	pound
Lg	large
mcg	microgram
med	medium
misc	miscellaneous
mg	milligram(s)
ml	milliliter
oz	ounce

pc	piece
pkg	package
pkt	packet
prep	prepared
sm	small
svg	serving
sq	square
Tbsp	tablespoon
Tr	trace—less than 1 g or mg
tsp	teaspoon
w/	with
w/o	without

Please Note

- All listings are medium- or average-portion size, unless specifically noted.

- "Cooked" means the food is cooked without added fats, sauces, or sugars. This includes boiling, steaming, and heating in a microwave oven.

- "Baked" and "broiled" describe the normal methods of baking and broiling, without oil, or minimal cooking oil for a non-stick surface. No other fats, sauces, or sugars have been added.

- Names in *italics* signify registered trademarks.

- Net carbs are taken from the manufacturers' nutritional information, or calculated by subtracting fiber from total cards. Net carbs are rounded to whole numbers.

- The data is accurate at the time publication. However, food manufacturers may change their ingredients at any time without notice. Food nutrition labels should also be checked. Keep your eyes open for new low-carb products!

References for Compiling This Book

- The United States Department of Agriculture (USDA), National Nutrient Database for Standard Reference, Release 21 (2008)

- Food manufacturers' nutrient labels (2009)

- Restaurants' printed nutritional data (2009)

BEVERAGES

	SERVING SIZE	CALORIES	TOTAL CARBS (g)	FIBER (g)	NET CARBS (g)	PROTEIN (g)	FAT (g)
Apple Juice, canned or bottled	8 fl oz	120	28	Tr	28	Tr	Tr
Apple juice, frozen concentrate (prepared)	8 fl oz	110	28	Tr	28	Tr	Tr
Apple-Cranberry Juice	8 fl oz	120	29	Tr	29	Tr	Tr
Apple-Grape Juice	8 fl oz	130	31	Tr	31	Tr	Tr
Apricot Nectar	8 fl oz	140	36	2	34	Tr	Tr
Beer	...	.	.	.	.	.	.
Regular Beer	12 fl oz	150	13	0	13	2	0
Light Beer	12 fl oz	100	6	0	6	Tr	0
Bourbon – see Distilled Spirits	...	...	.	.	.	.	.
Brandy – see Distilled Spirits	...	...	.	.	.	.	.
Capri Sun juice drink	8 fl oz	120	29	Tr	29	Tr	0
Carbonated Beverages – see Soda	...	...	.	.	.	.	.
Carrot Juice	8 fl oz	90	22	2	20	2	Tr
Club Soda – see Soda	...	...	.	.	.	.	.
Cocoa / Chocolate Beverage, Hot	...	...	.	.	.	.	.
Regular, as prep	6 fl oz	110	24	1	23	2	1
Diet or sugarfree, as prep	6 fl oz	60	11	1	10	2	Tr

	SERVING SIZE	CALORIES	TOTAL CARBS (g)	FIBER (g)	NET CARBS (g)	PROTEIN (g)	FAT (g)
Nestlé Rich Chocolate Hot Cocoa Mix	1 envelope	80	15	Tr	15	Tr	3
Nestlé Rich Chocolate Hot Cocoa Mix, with marshmallows	1 envelope	80	15	Tr	15	Tr	3
Ovaltine Sugar-Free Hot Cocoa	6 fl oz	40	7	Tr	7	3	Tr
Coffee	...	...	.	.	.	.	.
Brewed coffee, regular or decaf	6 fl oz	0	0	0	0	Tr	0
Instant coffee, regular or decaf	6 fl oz	0	Tr	0	Tr	Tr	0
Espresso	2 fl oz	0	0	0	0	Tr	Tr
Cappuccino, made w/ 4 oz milk	...	...	.	.	.	.	.
w/ whole milk (3.25%)	6 fl oz	80	6	0	6	4	4
w/ reduced fat milk (2%)	6 fl oz	60	6	0	6	4	2
w/ lowfat milk (1%)	6 fl oz	50	6	0	6	4	1
w/ nonfat milk	6 fl oz	45	6	0	6	4	Tr
Latte, made w/ 10 oz milk	...	...	.	.	.	.	.
w/ whole milk (3.25%)	12 fl oz	180	14	0	14	10	10
w/ reduced fat milk (2%)	12 fl oz	150	14	0	14	10	6
w/ lowfat milk (1%)	12 fl oz	130	15	0	15	10	3
w/ nonfat milk	12 fl oz	100	15	0	15	10	Tr

	SERVING SIZE	CALORIES	TOTAL CARBS (g)	FIBER (g)	NET CARBS (g)	PROTEIN (g)	FAT (g)
Cappuccino-flavored instant powder	4 tsp	50	11	Tr	11	Tr	Tr
French-flavored instant powder	4 tsp	60	9	0	9	Tr	3
Mocha-flavored instant powder	2 Tbsp	60	10	Tr	10	Tr	2
Coffee Cream – see Creamer	...	...	.	.	.	.	.
Coffee Liqueur, 53 proof	1.5 fl oz	170	24	0	24	Tr	Tr
Coke – see Soda	...	...	.	.	.	.	.
Cola – see Soda	...	...	.	.	.	.	.
Cranberry-Apple Juice Drink	8 fl oz	150	39	0	39	0	Tr
Cranberry Juice Cocktail, bottled	8 fl oz	140	34	0	34	0	Tr
Cranberry Juice Cocktail, frozen concentrate, as prep	8 fl oz	110	28	0	28	0	0
Cranberry-Grape Drink	8 fl oz	140	34	Tr	34	Tr	Tr
Cranberry-Apricot Juice Drink	8 fl oz	160	40	Tr	40	Tr	0
Cream Soda – see Soda	...	...	.	.	.	.	.
Creamer	.	.	.	.	.	.	.
Half & Half (cream & milk)	1 Tbsp	20	Tr	0	Tr	Tr	2
Half & Half (cream & milk)	1 cup	320	10	0	10	7	28
Half & Half, fat free	1 Tbsp	10	1	0	1	Tr	Tr
Coffee-Mate, Original liquid creamer	1 Tbsp	20	2	0	2	0	1

	SERVING SIZE	CALORIES	TOTAL CARBS (g)	FIBER (g)	NET CARBS (g)	PROTEIN (g)	FAT (g)
Coffee-Mate, Original powdered creamer	1 tsp	10	1	0	1	0	Tr
Liquid creamer	1 container	20	2	0	2	Tr	2
Liquid creamer, flavored	1 Tbsp	40	5	Tr	5	Tr	2
Liquid creamer, light	1 Tbsp	10	1	0	1	Tr	Tr
Powdered creamer	1 tsp	10	1	0	1	Tr	Tr
Powdered creamer, flavored	1 tsp	10	2	0	2	0	Tr
Powdered creamer, light	1 packet	15	2	0	2	Tr	Tr
SILK Original Creamer	1 Tbsp	15	1	0	1	0	1
Crème de Menthe	1.5 fl oz	190	21	0	21	0	Tr
Crystal Light, all flavors	8 fl oz	5	0	0	0	0	0
Daiquiri	2 fl oz	110	4	Tr	4	Tr	Tr
Diet Cola-see Soda	...	...	.	.	.	.	.
Diet Soda-see Soda	...	...	.	.	.	.	.
Distilled Spirits	...	...	.	.	.	.	.
80 proof	1.5 fl oz	100	0	0	0	0	0
86 proof	1.5 fl oz	110	Tr	0	Tr	0	0
90 proof	1.5 fl oz	110	0	0	0	0	0
Eggnog, plain	1 cup	340	34	0	34	10	19
Fruit Juice Drink, Citrus, frozen concentrate, as prep	8 fl oz	110	28	Tr	28	Tr	Tr

	SERVING SIZE	CALORIES	TOTAL CARBS (g)	FIBER (g)	NET CARBS (g)	PROTEIN (g)	FAT (g)
Fruit Punch Drink, frozen concentrate, as prep	8 fl oz	110	29	Tr	29	Tr	0
Fruit Punch Juice Drink, frozen concentrate, as prep	8 fl oz	100	24	0	24	Tr	Tr
Fruit-flavored drink mix, powdered, low calorie	1 tsp	5	2	0	2	0	0
Fruit-flavored drink mix, powdered, unsweetened	2 tsp	60	23	0	23	0	0
Gatorade	8 fl oz	50	14	0	14	0	0
Gin-see Distilled Spirits	...	...	.	.	.	.	.
Grape Juice, canned or bottled, unsweetened	8 fl oz	150	37	Tr	37	Tr	Tr
Grape Juice Cocktail, frozen concentrate, as prep	8 fl oz	130	32	Tr	32	Tr	Tr
Grapefruit Juice	...	...	.	.	.	.	.
Fresh squeezed	8 fl oz	100	23	Tr	23	1	Tr
Canned, unsweetened	8 fl oz	90	22	Tr	22	1	Tr
Canned, sugar sweetened	8 fl oz	120	28	Tr	28	2	Tr
Frozen concentrate, unsweetened, as prep w/ water	8 fl oz	100	24	Tr	24	1	Tr

	SERVING SIZE	CALORIES	TOTAL CARBS (g)	FIBER (g)	NET CARBS (g)	PROTEIN (g)	FAT (g)
Half & Half – see Creamer	...	...	.	.	.	.	.
Hawaiian Punch	...	...	.	.	.	.	.
Regular	8 fl oz	120	30	Tr	30	0	0
Light	8 fl oz	45	11	0	11	0	0
Hot Cocoa/ Chocolate – see	...	...	.	.	.	.	.
Cocoa	...	...	.	.	.	.	.
Juice – see specific listings	...	...	.	.	.	.	.
Kool Aid	...	...	.	.	.	.	.
Sugar sweetened	8 fl oz	60	16	Tr	16	0	0
Sugarfree	8 fl oz	5	0	0	0	0	0
Unsweetened Packet	1 pkt	0	0	0	0	0	0
Lemon Juice	...	...	.	.	.	.	.
Fresh squeezed	1 Tbsp	0	1	Tr	1	Tr	0
Fresh squeezed	1 cup	60	21	1	20	Tr	0
Canned or bottled, unsweetened	1 Tbsp	0	Tr	Tr	Tr	Tr	Tr
Canned or bottled, unsweetened	1 cup	50	16	1	15	Tr	Tr
Lemonade	...	...	.	.	.	.	.
Frozen concentrate, as prep (white or pink)	8 fl oz	100	26	Tr	26	Tr	Tr
Powdered, sugarfree, as prep	8 fl oz	5	2	0	2	Tr	0
Powdered, as prep	8 fl oz	100	26	0	26	0	0

	SERVING SIZE	CALORIES	TOTAL CARBS (g)	FIBER (g)	NET CARBS (g)	PROTEIN (g)	FAT (g)
Lemonade-flavor drink	...	...	.	.	.	.	.
Powdered, as prep	8 fl oz	70	17	0	17	Tr	0
Lime Juice	...	...	.	.	.	.	.
Canned or bottled, unsweetened	1 Tbsp	0	1	Tr	1	Tr	Tr
Canned or bottled, unsweetened	1 cup	50	17	1	16	Tr	Tr
Fresh squeezed	1 Tbsp	0	1	Tr	1	Tr	Tr
Fresh squeezed	1 cup	60	20	1	19	1	Tr
Limeade	...	...	.	.	.	.	.
Frozen concentrate, as prep	8 fl oz	130	34	0	34	0	0
Liqueur, 53 proof	1.5 fl oz	170	24	0	24	Tr	Tr
Liqueur, 63 proof	1.5 fl oz	160	17	0	17	Tr	Tr
Mai Tai	5 fl oz	280	28	1	27	1	Tr
Margarita	5 fl oz	150	10	Tr	10	0	0
Martini	2.5 fl oz	155	0	0	0	0	0
Milk	...	...	.	.	.	.	.
White Milk	...	...	.	.	.	.	.
Whole milk, 3.25% fat	8 fl oz	150	11	0	11	8	8
Reduced fat milk, 2% fat	8 fl oz	120	11	0	11	8	5
Lowfat milk, 1% fat	8 fl oz	100	12	0	12	8	2
Nonfat milk, (Skim milk)	8 fl oz	90	12	0	12	8	Tr
Nonfat instant, as prep w/ water	8 fl oz	80	12	0	12	8	Tr

	SERVING SIZE	CALORIES	TOTAL CARBS (g)	FIBER (g)	NET CARBS (g)	PROTEIN (g)	FAT (g)
Nonfat instant, dry powder only	1 cup	240	36	0	36	24	Tr
Chocolate Milk	. . .	. . .	.	.	.	.	.
Whole chocolate milk	8 fl oz	210	26	2	24	8	9
Reduced fat chocolate milk	8 fl oz	190	30	2	28	8	5
Lowfat chocolate milk	8 fl oz	160	26	1	25	8	3
Misc Milk Products	. . .	. . .	.	.	.	.	.
Buttermilk, lowfat	1 cup	100	12	0	12	8	2
Buttermilk, dried	1 Tbsp	25	3	0	3	2	Tr
Condensed, sweetened	1 cup	980	167	0	167	24	27
Evaporated skim milk	1 cup	200	29	0	29	19	Tr
Evaporated whole milk	1 cup	340	25	0	25	17	19
Malted milk, chocolate	1 cup	225	30	1	29	9	9
Malted milk, natural	1 cup	230	27	Tr	27	10	10
Saco Cultured Buttermilk Blend, powdered	4 Tbsp	80	13	0	13	5	Tr
Soymilk	. . .	. . .	.	.	.	.	.
Unsweetened	1 cup	80	4	1	3	7	4
Vanilla	1 cup	100	12	Tr	12	6	4
Chocolate	1 cup	150	24	1	23	6	4

	SERVING SIZE	CALORIES	TOTAL CARBS (g)	FIBER (g)	NET CARBS (g)	PROTEIN (g)	FAT (g)
Vitasoy Organic Classic Original Soymilk	1 cup	45	5	Tr	5	3	2
Vitasoy Light Vanilla Soymilk	1 cup	70	10	Tr	10	4	2
SILK, unsweetened soymilk	1 cup	80	4	1	3	7	4
SILK, vanilla soymilk	1 cup	100	10	1	9	6	4
SILK, chocolate soymilk	1 cup	140	23	2	21	5	4
Milk Shake – see Shake	...	...	.	.	.	.	.
Nesquik	...	...	.	.	.	.	.
Chocolate Syrup	1 Tbsp	70	16	0	16	0	0
Chocolate Syrup, ⅓ less sugar	1 Tbsp	50	10	0	10	0	0
Vanilla, ⅓ less sugar	1 Tbsp	50	12	0	12	0	0
Strawberry, ⅓ less sugar	1 Tbsp	50	11	1	10	0	0
Orange Juice	...	...	.	.	.	.	.
Fresh squeezed	8 fl oz	110	26	Tr	26	2	Tr
Canned, unsweetened	8 fl oz	120	27	Tr	27	2	Tr
Chilled, from concentrate	8 fl oz	110	25	Tr	25	2	Tr
Frozen concentrate, as prep	8 fl oz	110	27	Tr	27	2	Tr
Peach Nectar	8 fl oz	130	35	2	33	Tr	Tr
Pear Nectar	8 fl oz	150	39	2	37	Tr	Tr
Pepsi – see Soda	...	...	.	.	.	.	.
Pina Colada	4.5 fl oz	250	32	Tr	32	Tr	3

	SERVING SIZE	CALORIES	TOTAL CARBS (g)	FIBER (g)	NET CARBS (g)	PROTEIN (g)	FAT (g)
Pineapple Grapefruit Juice	8 fl oz	120	29	Tr	29	Tr	Tr
Pineapple Juice	...	...	.	.	.	.	.
Canned, unsweetened	8 fl oz	130	32	Tr	32	Tr	Tr
Frozen concentrate, as prep	8 fl oz	130	32	Tr	32	1	Tr
Pineapple Orange Juice	8 fl oz	125	30	Tr	30	3	0
Powerade, Lemon-lime flavored	8 fl oz	80	19	0	19	0	Tr
Propel Fitness Water, fruit-flavored	8 fl oz	10	3	0	3	0	0
Prune Juice	8 fl oz	180	45	3	42	2	Tr
Root Beer – see Soda	...	...	.	.	.	.	.
Rum–see Distilled Spirits	...	...	.	.	.	.	.
Sake (rice wine)	1 fl oz	40	2	0	2	Tr	0
Scotch-see Distilled Spirits	...	...	.	.	.	.	.
Screwdriver	7 fl oz	160	17	1	16	Tr	Tr
Shake	...	...	.	.	.	.	.
Regular milk shake	...	...	.	.	.	.	.
Chocolate	11 oz	370	66	Tr	66	10	8
Vanilla	11 oz	350	56	0	56	12	10
Atkins Advantage low carb shake	...	...	.	.	.	.	.
Café Caramel Shake	11 oz	160	3	2	1	15	9
Chocolate Royale Shake	11 oz	160	5	4	1	15	9

	SERVING SIZE	CALORIES	TOTAL CARBS (g)	FIBER (g)	NET CARBS (g)	PROTEIN (g)	FAT (g)
Milk Chocolate Delight Shake	11 oz	160	4	3	1	15	9
Mocha Latte Shake	11 oz	160	5	3	2	15	9
Strawberry Shake	11 oz	150	2	2	0	15	9
Vanilla Shake	11 oz	150	2	2	0	15	9
Soda / Cola / Soft Drink	...	...	.	.	.	.	.
(Carbonated Beverages)	...	...	.	.	.	.	.
Barq's Root Beer	12 fl oz	170	45	0	45	0	0
Barq's Root Beer, diet	12 fl oz	0	Tr	0	Tr	0	0
Cherry Coke	12 fl oz	160	42	0	42	0	0
Cherry Coke, diet	12 fl oz	0	Tr	0	Tr	0	0
Club Soda	12 fl oz	0	0	0	0	0	0
Coca-Cola Classic	12 fl oz	150	41	0	41	0	0
Coke, diet	12 fl oz	0	Tr	0	Tr	0	0
Cola	12 fl oz	140	35	0	35	Tr	Tr
Cola, no caffeine	12 fl oz	150	39	0	39	0	0
Cream Soda	12 fl oz	190	49	0	49	0	0
Diet Cola, with aspartame	12 fl oz	5	1	0	1	Tr	Tr
Diet Cola, with sodium saccharin	12 fl oz	0	Tr	0	Tr	0	0
Dr Pepper, diet	12 fl oz	0	0	0	0	0	0
Dr Pepper, regular	12 fl oz	150	41	0	41	0	0

	SERVING SIZE	CALORIES	TOTAL CARBS (g)	FIBER (g)	NET CARBS (g)	PROTEIN (g)	FAT (g)
Fresca	12 fl oz	0	Tr	0	Tr	0	0
Ginger Ale, regular	12 fl oz	120	32	0	32	0	0
Grape Soda, regular	12 fl oz	160	42	0	42	0	0
Lemon Lime Soda, regular	12 fl oz	150	39	0	39	Tr	0
Mountain Dew, diet	12 fl oz	0	0	0	0	0	0
Mountain Dew, regular	12 fl oz	170	46	0	46	0	0
Mug Cream Soda	12 fl oz	180	47	0	47	0	0
Mug Cream Soda, diet	12 fl oz	0	0	0	0	0	0
Mug Root Beer	12 fl oz	160	43	0	43	0	0
Mug Root Beer, Diet	12 fl oz	0	0	0	0	0	0
Orange Soda, regular	12 fl oz	180	46	0	46	0	0
Pepsi Max	12 fl oz	0	0	0	0	0	0
Pepsi One	12 fl oz	0	0	0	0	0	0
Pepsi, diet	12 fl oz	0	0	0	0	0	0
Pepsi, regular and caffeine free	12 fl oz	150	41	0	41	0	0
Pibb Xtra	12 fl oz	150	39	0	39	0	0
Pibb Zero	12 fl oz	0	Tr	0	Tr	0	0
RC Cola, diet	12 fl oz	0	0	0	0	0	0
RC Cola, regular	12 fl oz	160	43	0	43	0	0
Root Beer, Regular	12 fl oz	150	39	0	39	0	0
Seven Up, diet	12 fl oz	0	0	0	0	0	0
Seven Up, regular	12 fl oz	150	39	0	39	0	0

	SERVING SIZE	CALORIES	TOTAL CARBS (g)	FIBER (g)	NET CARBS (g)	PROTEIN (g)	FAT (g)
Sierra Mist	12 fl oz	140	39	0	39	0	0
Sierra Mist, Diet	12 fl oz	0	0	0	0	0	0
Sprite Zero	12 fl oz	0	0	0	0	0	0
Sprite, regular	12 fl oz	150	37	0	37	Tr	0
Tab	12 fl oz	0	Tr	0	Tr	0	0
Tonic water	12 fl oz	120	32	0	32	0	0
Soft Drinks – see Soda	...	...	.		.	.	.
Sport Drink – see specific listings	...	...	.		.	.	.
Sugarfree Beverage–see specific listings	...	.	.		.	.	.
SunnyD	...	...	.		.	.	.
Fruit Punch	8 fl oz	80	21	Tr	21	0	0
Mango	8 fl oz	90	22	Tr	22	0	0
Smooth Style	8 fl oz	90	22	Tr	22	0	0
Tangy Original Style	8 fl oz	90	22	Tr	22	0	0
SunnyD with calcium	8 fl oz	140	35	Tr	35	0	0
SunnyD Reduced Sugar	8 fl oz	60	15	Tr	15	0	0
Tang	...	...	.	.	.	.	.
Regular	8 fl oz	115	29	Tr	29	0	0
Sugarfree	8 fl oz	5	0	0	0	0	0
Tangerine Juice, fresh squeezed	8 fl oz	110	25	Tr	25	1	Tr
Tea	...	...	.	.	.	.	.
Regular, Decaf, or Herbal	...	...	.	.	.	.	.
unsweetened	8 fl oz	0	Tr	0	Tr	0	0

	SERVING SIZE	CALORIES	TOTAL CARBS (g)	FIBER (g)	NET CARBS (g)	PROTEIN (g)	FAT (g)
sweetened with 1 teaspoon sugar	8 fl oz	20	5	0	5	0	0
sweetened with 1 packet aspartame	8 fl oz	5	2	0	2	Tr	0
Instant	. . .	. . .	.	.	.	.	.
unsweetened	8 fl oz	0	Tr	0	Tr	Tr	0
sweetened with sugar, lemon-flavored	8 fl oz	90	22	Tr	22	Tr	Tr
sweetened with sodium saccharin, lemon-flavored	8 fl oz	5	1	0	1	Tr	0
Arizona iced tea, lemon flavor	8 fl oz	90	22	0	22	0	0
Lipton Brisk iced tea, lemon flavor	8 fl oz	90	22	0	22	0	0
Nestle Cool Nestea ice tea, lemon flavor	8 fl oz	90	22	0	22	0	0
Tequila	1.5 fl oz	100	0	0	0	0	0
Tequila Sunrise	5.5 fl oz	190	19	0	19	Tr	Tr
Tomato Juice, canned	8 fl oz	40	10	1	9	2	Tr
Tomato & Clam Juice, canned	8 fl oz	120	27	1	26	2	Tr
Tonic Water-see Soda	. . .	. . .	.	.	.	.	.
V8 SPLASH **Juice Drinks**	. . .	. . .	.	.	.	.	.

	SERVING SIZE	CALORIES	TOTAL CARBS (g)	FIBER (g)	NET CARBS (g)	PROTEIN (g)	FAT (g)
Berry Blend, Orange Pineapple, Strawberry Banana, Strawberry Kiwi, Tropical Blend	8 fl oz	70	18	0	18	0	0
Fruit Medley, Guava Passion Fruit, Orchard Blend	8 fl oz	80	19	0	19	0	0
Mango Peach	8 fl oz	80	20	0	20	0	0
V8 SPLASH Juice Drinks, All Diet Blends	8 fl oz	10	3	0	3	0	0
V* SPLASH Smoothies	...	...	.	.	.	.	.
Peach Mango	8 fl oz	90	19	0	19	3	0
Strawberry Banana	8 fl oz	90	20	0	20	3	0
Tropical Colada	8 fl oz	100	21	1	20	3	0
V8 Vegetable Juice	8 fl oz	50	10	2	8	2	0
Vegetable Juice	8 fl oz	45	11	2	9	2	Tr
Vodka-see Distilled Spirits	...	...	.	.	.	.	.
Water	8 fl oz	0	0	0	0	0	0
Whiskey-see Distilled Spirits	...	...	.	.	.	.	.
Wine	...	...	.	.	.	.	.
Cooking wine	1 fl oz	15	2	0	2	Tr	0
Dessert Wine, Dry	3.5 fl oz	150	12	0	12	Tr	0

	SERVING SIZE	CALORIES	TOTAL CARBS (g)	FIBER (g)	NET CARBS (g)	PROTEIN (g)	FAT (g)
Dessert Wine, Sweet	3.2 fl oz	170	14	0	14	Tr	0
Non-alcoholic Wine	5 fl oz	10	2	0	2	Tr	0
Red Wine (table wine)	5 fl oz	130	4	0	4	Tr	0
Rice Wine-see Sake	...	...	.	.	.	.	.
Rosè Wine	5 fl oz	120	4	0	4	Tr	0
White Wine (table wine)	5 fl oz	120	4	0	4	Tr	0
White Zinfandel	5 fl oz	120	4	0	4	Tr	0

FOODS

	SERVING SIZE	CALORIES	TOTAL CARBS (g)	FIBER (g)	NET CARBS (g)	PROTEIN (g)	FAT (g)
Alfalfa sprouts, fresh	1 cup	10	Tr	Tr	Tr	1	Tr
Almonds – see Nuts	…	…	.	.	.	.	.
Anchovy – see Fish	…	…	.	.	.	.	.
Anise Seed	1 Tbsp	25	3	1	2	1	1
Apple	…	…	.	.	.	.	.
Fresh, unpeeled, sm 2¾″ dia	1	80	21	4	17	Tr	Tr
Fresh, unpeeled, med 3″ dia	1	100	25	4	21	Tr	Tr
Fresh, peeled, sliced	1 cup	50	14	1	13	Tr	Tr
Dried	5 rings	80	21	3	18	Tr	Tr
Apple Butter	1 Tbsp	30	7	Tr	7	Tr	Tr
Apple Pie Filling, 1 portion	2⅔ oz	80	20	Tr	20	Tr	Tr
Applesauce	…	…	.	.	.	.	.
Sweetened	½ cup	100	25	2	23	Tr	Tr
Unsweetened	½ cup	50	14	2	12	Tr	Tr
Apricot	…	…	.	.	.	.	.
Fresh, medium size, 1.3 oz	1	15	4	1	3	Tr	Tr
Canned halves, in heavy syrup	1 cup	220	55	4	51	1	Tr
Canned halves, in juice	1 cup	120	30	4	26	2	Tr
Dried, halves	10 halves	90	22	3	19	1	Tr
Artichoke, Globe or French	…	…	.	.	.	.	.
Fresh, cooked med whole	1	60	14	10	4	4	Tr
Fresh, cooked hearts, drained	½ cup	45	10	7	3	2	Tr

	SERVING SIZE	CALORIES	TOTAL CARBS (g)	FIBER (g)	NET CARBS (g)	PROTEIN (g)	FAT (g)
Frozen, thawed and cooked	½ cup	40	8	4	4	3	Tr
Jerusalem artichoke, raw, sliced	1 cup	110	26	2	24	3	Tr
Arugula, raw	½ cup	0	Tr	Tr	Tr	Tr	Tr
Asparagus, cooked	. . .	.	.	.	.	.	.
Fresh, medium size spears	4 spears	15	3	1	2	1	Tr
Fresh, chopped pieces	½ cup	20	4	2	2	2	Tr
Frozen, spears	4 spears	10	1	1	0	2	Tr
Frozen, chopped pieces	1 cup	30	4	3	1	5	Tr
Canned, 5" spears	4 spears	15	2	1	1*	2	Tr
Canned, chopped pieces	1 cup	45	6	4	2*	5	2
Aspartame Sweetener (*Equal*)	1 pkt	0	Tr	0	Tr	Tr	0
Aspartame Sweetener (*Equal*)	1 tsp	15	3	0	3	Tr	0
Avocado	. . .	. . .	.	.	.	.	.
California, ⅕ of whole	1 oz	45	3	2	1	Tr	4
Florida, ⅒ of whole	1 oz	35	2	2	0	Tr	3
Bacon – see Pork	. . .	. . .	.	.	.	.	.
Bacon Bits	1 Tbsp	35	2	Tr	1	2	2
Bagel, med, 3¾ oz	. . .	. . .	.	.	.	.	.
Cinnamon raisin	1	290	58	2	56	10	2
Egg	1	290	56	2	54	11	2
Oatbran	1	270	56	4	52	11	1
Onion	1	290	56	2	54	11	2
Plain	1	290	56	2	54	11	2
Poppyseed	1	290	56	2	54	11	2
Sesame	1	290	56	2	54	11	2
Baking Powder	1 tsp	0	1	0	1	0	0

	SERVING SIZE	CALORIES	TOTAL CARBS (g)	FIBER (g)	NET CARBS (g)	PROTEIN (g)	FAT (g)
Baking Soda	1 tsp	0	0	0	0	0	0
Bamboo Shoots, canned, drained	1 cup	25	4	2	2	2	Tr
Banana	...	...	.	.	.	.	.
Fresh, 7" long	1	110	27	3	24	1	Tr
Fresh, sliced	1 cup	130	34	4	30	2	Tr
Barley, pearled, cooked	1 cup	190	44	6	38	4	Tr
Basil	...	...	.	.	.	.	.
Dried spice	1 tsp	0	Tr	Tr	Tr	Tr	Tr
Fresh, chopped	2 Tbsp	0	Tr	Tr	Tr	Tr	Tr
Fresh, whole leaves	¼ cup	0	Tr	Tr	Tr	Tr	Tr
Bean Sprouts (mung)	...	...	.	.	.	.	.
Cooked, boiled	1 cup	25	5	1	4	3	Tr
Cooked, stir-fried	1 cup	60	13	2	11	5	Tr
Fresh	1 cup	30	6	2	4	3	Tr
BEANS	...	...	.	.	.	.	.
Plain Beans, cooked w/o fats	...	...	.	.	.	.	.
Adzuki beans	½ cup	150	29	8	21	9	Tr
Black beans	½ cup	110	20	8	12	8	Tr
Chickpeas (garbanzo beans)	½ cup	130	23	6	17	7	2
Cranberry (roman) beans	½ cup	120	22	9	13	8	Tr
Fava beans(broadbeans)	½ cup	90	17	5	12	7	Tr
Great Northern beans	½ cup	100	19	6	13	7	Tr
Kidney, Red beans	½ cup	110	20	7	13	8	Tr
Lima, baby lima beans	½ cup	120	21	7	14	7	Tr
Lima, large beans	½ cup	110	20	7	13	7	Tr
Navy beans	½ cup	130	24	10	14	8	Tr

	SERVING SIZE	CALORIES	TOTAL CARBS (g)	FIBER (g)	NET CARBS (g)	PROTEIN (g)	FAT (g)
Pinto beans	½ cup	120	22	8	14	8	Tr
Soybeans	½ cup	150	9	5	4	14	8
White beans	½ cup	120	23	6	17	9	Tr
Snap Beans (stringbeans), cooked w/o fats	...	...	.	.	.	.	.
Canned, drained	1 cup	25	6	3	3	2	Tr
Green beans, fresh	1 cup	45	10	4	6	2	Tr
Frozen, cooked	1 cup	40	9	4	5	2	Tr
Yellow (wax) beans, fresh	1 cup	45	10	4	6	2	Tr
Misc Bean Dishes, as prep	...	...	.	.	.	.	.
Baked beans, plain or vegetarian	½ cup	120	27	5	22	6	Tr
Baked beans w/ frankfurters	½ cup	180	20	9	11	9	9
Baked beans w/ pork	½ cup	130	25	7	18	7	2
Baked beans w/pork and tomato sauce	½ cup	120	23	5	18	6	1
Baked beans w/pork and sweet sauce	½ cup	140	27	5	22	7	2
Campbell's Brown Sugar and Bacon Flavored Beans	½ cup	160	30	8	22	5	3
Campbell's Pork and Beans	½ cup	140	25	7	18	6	2
Refried beans	½ cup	110	18	6	12	6	1
Refried beans, fat-free	½ cup	90	16	5	11	6	Tr
Refried red beans	½ cup	170	18	6	12	6	8
Refried beans, vegetarian	½ cup	100	16	6	10	6	1

	SERVING SIZE	CALORIES	TOTAL CARBS (g)	FIBER (g)	NET CARBS (g)	PROTEIN (g)	FAT (g)
BEEF	...	...	.	.	.	.	.
(Weights for meat w/o bones)	...	...	.	.	.	.	.
(Meats trimmed to 0% fat, unless otherwise noted)	...	...	.	.	.	.	.
Bottom Round, braised	...	...	.	.	.	.	.
lean & fat	3 oz	190	0	0	0	29	8
lean only	3 oz	180	0	0	0	29	7
Brisket, braised	...	...	.	.	.	.	.
flat half, lean & fat	3 oz	180	0	0	0	28	7
flat half, lean only	3 oz	170	0	0	0	28	6
point half, lean & fat	3 oz	300	0	0	0	20	24
point half, lean only	3 oz	210	0	0	0	24	12
whole, lean & fat	3 oz	250	0	0	0	23	17
whole, lean only	3 oz	190	0	0	0	25	9
Chuck Blade, Blade Roast, braised	...	...	.	.	.	.	.
lean & fat	3 oz	300	0	0	0	23	22
lean only	3 oz	220	0	0	0	26	11
Chuck, Top Blade, broiled	...	...	.	.	.	.	.
lean & fat	3 oz	180	0	0	0	22	10
lean only	3 oz	170	0	0	0	22	9
Corned Beef	3 oz	210	0	0	0	23	13
Dried Beef, chipped	1 oz	45	Tr	0	Tr	9	Tr
Eye of Round, roasted	...	...	.	.	.	.	.
lean & fat	3 oz	140	0	0	0	25	4
lean only	3 oz	140	0	0	0	25	4
Flank Steak, broiled	...	...	.	.	.	.	.
lean & fat	3 oz	160	0	0	0	24	7
lean only	3 oz	160	0	0	0	24	6

	SERVING SIZE	CALORIES	TOTAL CARBS (g)	FIBER (g)	NET CARBS (g)	PROTEIN (g)	FAT (g)
Ground Beef / Hamburger meat, broiled	...	...	.	.	.	.	.
75% lean meat	3 oz	240	0	0	0	22	16
80% lean meat	3 oz	230	0	0	0	22	15
85% lean meat	3 oz	210	0	0	0	22	13
90% lean meat	3 oz	180	0	0	0	22	10
Liver, fried	3 oz	150	4	0	4	23	4
Pastrami	2 oz	80	0	0	0	12	3
Porterhouse Steak, broiled	...	...	.	.	.	.	.
lean & fat	3 oz	240	0	0	0	20	16
lean only	3 oz	180	0	0	0	22	10
Pot Roast, Chuck, braised	...	...	.	.	.	.	.
lean & fat	3 oz	250	0	0	0	25	16
lean only	3 oz	170	0	0	0	28	5
Prime Rib (trimmed to ⅛" fat), broiled	3 oz	330	0	0	0	19	28
Rib Roast (trimmed to ⅛" fat), roasted	3 oz	300	0	0	0	19	24
Roast Beef, sliced deli meat	2 oz	70	2	0	2	10	2
Short Ribs, braised	...	...	.	.	.	.	.
lean & fat	3 oz	400	0	0	0	18	36
lean only	3 oz	250	0	0	0	26	15
Top Sirloin, broiled	...	...	.	.	.	.	.
lean & fat	3 oz	180	0	0	0	25	8
lean only	3 oz	160	0	0	0	26	5
T-bone Steak, broiled	...	...	.	.	.	.	.
lean & fat	3 oz	210	0	0	0	21	14
lean only	3 oz	160	0	0	0	22	7

	SERVING SIZE	CALORIES	TOTAL CARBS (g)	FIBER (g)	NET CARBS (g)	PROTEIN (g)	FAT (g)
Tenderloin Steak, broiled	...	...	.	.	.	.	.
lean & fat	3 oz	190	0	0	0	23	10
lean only	3 oz	160	0	0	0	24	7
Top Round, braised	...	...	.	.	.	.	.
lean & fat	3 oz	180	0	0	0	30	6
lean only	3 oz	170	0	0	0	31	4
Tri-tip Steak, broiled	...	...	.	.	.	.	.
lean & fat	3 oz	230	0	0	0	26	13
lean only	3 oz	210	0	0	0	26	11
(Other Beef Products, see:	...	...	.	.	.	.	.
Bologna, Hot Dog, Salami,	...	...	.	.	.	.	.
Sausage & specific entrées)	...	...	.	.	.	.	.
Beef Macaroni, frozen entree	8.5 oz	210	34	5	29	14	2
Beef Jerky	1 piece	80	2	Tr	2	7	5
Beef Stew, Dinty Moore, canned	1 cup	220	16	3	13	11	13
Beet Greens, chopped, cooked	½ cup	20	4	2	2*	2	Tr
Beets	...	...	.	.	.	.	.
Fresh, cooked, slices	½ cup	35	9	2	7	1	Tr
Fresh, cooked, whole, 2" dia	2	45	10	2	8	2	Tr
Canned, drained, slices	½ cup	25	6	2	4	Tr	Tr
Canned, drained, whole	1 cup	50	12	3	9	2	Tr
Canned, pickled, slices with liquid	½ cup	70	19	3	16	Tr	Tr
Biscuit, plain or buttermilk	...	...	.	.	.	.	.

	SERVING SIZE	CALORIES	TOTAL CARBS (g)	FIBER (g)	NET CARBS (g)	PROTEIN (g)	FAT (g)
Prep from recipe, 2 ½" dia	1	210	27	1	26	4	10
Prep from recipe, 4" dia	1	360	45	2	43	7	17
Refrigerated dough, baked	...	...	.	.	.	.	.
regular 2 ½" dia	1	100	13	Tr	13	2	4
reduced fat, 2 ¼" dia	1	60	12	Tr	12	2	1
Blackberries	...	...	.	.	.	.	.
Fresh	1 cup	60	14	8	6	2	Tr
Frozen, unthawed	1 cup	100	24	8	16	2	Tr
Blueberries	...	...	.	.	.	.	.
Fresh	1 cup	80	22	4	18	1	Tr
Frozen, sweetened, thawed	1 cup	190	51	5	46	Tr	Tr
Frozen, unsweetened, unthawed	1 cup	80	19	4	15	Tr	Tr
Frozen, wild, unthawed	1 cup	70	19	6	13	0	Tr
Bologna	...	...	.	.	.	.	.
Beef	1 slice	90	1	0	1	3	8
Beef, lowfat	1 slice	60	2	0	2	3	4
Beef & Pork	1 slice	90	2	0	2	4	7
Beef & Pork, lowfat	1 slice	60	Tr	0	Tr	3	5
Boars Head, Beef & Pork	2 oz	150	1	0	1	7	13
Louis Rich, Turkey Bologna	1 slice	50	1	0	1	3	4
Oscar Mayer, Beef Light	1 slice	60	2	0	2	3	4
Oscar Mayer, Bologna	1 slice	90	Tr	0	Tr	3	8
Oscar Mayer, Bologna, fat free	1 slice	20	2	0	2	4	Tr
Turkey	1 slice	60	1	Tr	1	3	5

	SERVING SIZE	CALORIES	TOTAL CARBS (g)	FIBER (g)	NET CARBS (g)	PROTEIN (g)	FAT (g)
Bouillon – see Soup	. . .	. . .	.	.	.	.	.
Bratwurst, *Boars Head*	1 wurst	300	0	0	0	19	25
Braunschweiger, Oscar Mayer brand, 1 slice	1 oz	90	Tr	Tr	Tr	4	8
BREAD	. . .	. . .	.	.	.	.	.
(avg ½" thick slice unless noted)	. . .	. . .	.	.	.	.	.
Boston brown, canned	1 slice	90	20	2	18	2	Tr
Cornbread, 3" × 2"	1 piece	190	29	1	28	4	6
Cracked Wheat	1 slice	80	15	2	13	3	1
Croissant	1 med	230	26	2	24	5	12
Croissant, apple	1 med	150	21	1	20	4	5
Croissant, cheese	1 med	240	27	2	25	5	12
Egg bread	1 slice	110	19	Tr	19	4	2
English muffin, cinnamon/raisin	1 whole	140	27	2	25	5	1
English muffin, mixed-grain	1 whole	160	31	2	29	6	1
English muffin, regular	1 whole	130	25	2	23	5	Tr
English muffin, whole-wheat	1 whole	130	27	4	23	6	1
French bread	1 slice	90	18	Tr	18	4	Tr
Garlic bread, Pepperidge Farm brand, frozen	1 slice	170	24	2	22	4	7
Irish soda bread	1 oz	80	16	Tr	16	2	1
Italian bread	1 slice	50	10	Tr	10	2	Tr
Multigrain bread	1 slice	70	11	2	9	4	1
Oat bread	1 slice	70	12	1	11	3	1
Oatmeal bread	1 slice	70	13	1	12	2	1
Pita bread, 4"	1 whole	80	16	Tr	16	3	Tr
Pita bread, 6 ½"	1 whole	170	33	1	32	5	Tr
Pita bread, whole-wheat, 4"	1 whole	70	15	2	13	3	Tr

	SERVING SIZE	CALORIES	TOTAL CARBS (g)	FIBER (g)	NET CARBS (g)	PROTEIN (g)	FAT (g)
Pita bread, whole-wheat, 6 ½″	1 whole	170	35	5	30	6	2
Pumpernickel bread	1 slice	80	15	2	13	3	1
Raisin bread	1 slice	90	17	1	16	3	1
Reduced calorie bread, white	1 slice	50	10	2	8	2	Tr
Ricebran bread	1 slice	70	12	1	11	2	1
Roll, dinner (egg)	1 roll	110	18	1	17	3	2
Roll, french	1 roll	110	19	1	18	3	2
Roll, hard or kaiser	1 roll	170	30	1	29	6	3
Roll, hamburger or hotdog	1 roll	120	21	Tr	21	4	2
Roll, hamburger or hotdog, mixed-grain	1 roll	110	19	2	17	4	3
Roll hamburger or hotdog, low cal	1 roll	80	18	3	15	4	Tr
Roll, whole-wheat	1 roll	100	18	3	15	3	2
Rye bread	1 slice	80	16	2	14	3	1
Sourdough bread	1 slice	90	18	Tr	18	4	Tr
Vienna bread	1 slice	90	18	Tr	18	4	Tr
Wheat bread	1 slice	70	12	Tr	12	3	Tr
White bread	1 slice	70	13	Tr	13	2	Tr
Whole-wheat bread	1 slice	70	12	2	10	4	Tr
(also see Bagel & Biscuit)	...	...	.	.	.	.	.
Bread Crumbs	...	...	.	.	.	.	.
Dry, grated	1 cup	430	78	5	73	14	6
Dry, seasoned, grated	1 cup	460	82	6	76	17	7
Panko Bread Crumbs, Ian's	¼ cup	70	15	Tr	15	2	0
Panko Japanese Style Bread Crumbs, Dynasty	½ cup	110	20	1	19	4	1
Soft crumbs	1 cup	120	23	1	22	3	2

	SERVING SIZE	CALORIES	TOTAL CARBS (g)	FIBER (g)	NET CARBS (g)	PROTEIN (g)	FAT (g)
Bread Stick, med	1	40	7	Tr	7	1	Tr
Bread Stuffing – see Stuffing	...	...	.	.	.	.	.
Breakfast Bar, w/oats, raisins, & coconut	1 bar	200	29	1	28	4	8
Breakfast Sandwich	...	...	.	.	.	.	.
Biscuit w/ Egg	1	370	32	Tr	32	12	22
Biscuit w/ Egg & Bacon	1	460	29	Tr	29	17	31
Biscuit w/ Egg, Bacon, & Cheese	1	440	35	Tr	35	17	25
Biscuit w/ Ham	1	440	31	Tr	31	20	27
Biscuit w/ Egg & Sausage	1	510	34	Tr	34	18	34
Biscuit w/ Ham	1	390	44	Tr	44	13	18
Biscuit w/ Sausage	1	410	33	Tr	33	11	27
Croissant w/ Egg & Cheese	1	370	24	Tr	24	13	25
Croissant w/ Egg, Cheese, & Bacon	1	410	24	Tr	24	16	28
Croissant w/ Egg, Cheese, & Ham	1	470	24	Tr	24	19	34
Croissant w/ Egg, Cheese, & Sausage	1	520	25	Tr	25	20	38
English Muffin w/ Egg, Cheese, & Canadian Bacon	1	310	30	Tr	30	19	13
English Muffin w/ Egg, Cheese, & Sausage	1	470	29	Tr	29	22	30
Broccoli	...	...	.	.	.	.	.
Fresh, raw, spear, 5" long	1	10	2	Tr	2	Tr	Tr
Fresh, raw, chopped	1 cup	30	6	2	4	3	Tr
Fresh, cooked, spear, 5" long	1	10	3	1	2	Tr	Tr

	SERVING SIZE	CALORIES	TOTAL CARBS (g)	FIBER (g)	NET CARBS (g)	PROTEIN (g)	FAT (g)
Fresh, chopped, cooked	½ cup	25	6	3	3	2	Tr
Frozen, chopped, cooked	1 cup	50	10	6	4	6	Tr
Frozen, spears, cooked	½ cup	25	5	3	2	3	Tr
Broccoli, Chinese, cooked	1 cup	20	3	3	1	1	Tr
Broccoli Rabe, cooked	3 oz	30	3	2	1	3	Tr
raw, chopped	1 cup	10	1	1	0	1	Tr
Broth – see Soup	...	...	.	.	.	.	.
Brownie, 2″ square	1	240	39	Tr	39	3	10
Brussels Sprouts	...	...	.	.	.	.	.
Fresh, cooked	1 cup	60	11	4	7	4	Tr
Frozen, cooked	1 cup	70	13	6	7	6	Tr
Bulgur	...	...	.	.	.	.	.
Cooked	1 cup	150	34	8	26	6	Tr
Uncooked	1 cup	480	106	26	80	17	2
Bun – see Bread, roll	...	...	.	.	.	.	.
Burrito	...	...	.	.	.	.	.
Bean & cheese	1	310	48	12	36	10	9
Beef & bean	1	350	45	8	37	10	14
Butter (also see margarine)	...	...	.	.	.	.	.
Regular, salted or unsalted, 1 stick	8 Tbsp	810	Tr	0	Tr	Tr	92
Regular, salted or unsalted	1 Tbsp	100	Tr	0	Tr	Tr	12
Regular, salted or unsalted	1 tsp	35	0	0	0	Tr	4
Cabbage	...	...	.	.	.	.	.
Green, raw, shredded	1 cup	15	4	2	2	Tr	Tr
Green, shredded, cooked	½ cup	15	4	1	3	Tr	Tr

	SERVING SIZE	CALORIES	TOTAL CARBS (g)	FIBER (g)	NET CARBS (g)	PROTEIN (g)	FAT (g)
Chinese cabbage (bok choy)	...	...	.	.	.	.	.
shredded, raw	1 cup	10	2	Tr	2	1	Tr
shredded, cooked	1 cup	20	3	2	1	3	Tr
Napa cabbage	1 cup	15	2	Tr	2	1	Tr
Red cabbage, raw, shredded	1 cup	20	5	2	3	1	Tr
Red cabbage, shredded, cooked	1 cup	45	10	4	6	2	Tr
Savoy cabbage, raw, shredded	1 cup	20	4	2	2	1	Tr
Savoy cabbage, shredded, cooked	1 cup	35	8	4	4	3	Tr
CAKE	...	...	.	.	.	.	.
(average size slice of single layer	...	...	.	.	.	.	.
cake, ⅛ of 9", unless noted)	...	.	.	.	.	.	.
Angelfood cake, ¹⁄₁₂ of 10" cake	1 piece	130	29	Tr	29	3	Tr
Boston Cream Cake, ⅛ of cake	1 piece	230	40	1	39	2	8
Cheesecake, ⅙ of 17 oz cake	1 piece	260	20	Tr	20	4	18
Chocolate cake w/ chocolate frosting	1 piece	240	35	2	33	3	11
Fruitcake, small slice	1 piece	140	27	2	25	1	4
Gingerbread	1 piece	260	36	1	35	3	12
Pineapple Upside Down Cake	1 piece	370	58	Tr	58	4	14
Pound Cake w/o glaze, ¹⁄₁₀ of cake	1 piece	120	15	Tr	15	2	6
Pound Cake, fat free, ¹⁄₁₀ of cake	1 piece	100	21	Tr	21	2	Tr
Sponge Cake, ¹⁄₁₀ of 10" cake	1 piece	110	23	Tr	23	2	1

	SERVING SIZE	CALORIES	TOTAL CARBS (g)	FIBER (g)	NET CARBS (g)	PROTEIN (g)	FAT (g)
White Cake, ½₂ of cake	...	...	.	.	.	.	.
w/coconut frosting	1 piece	400	71	1	70	5	12
w/o frosting	1 piece	260	42	Tr	42	4	9
Yellow Cake	...	...	.	.	.	.	.
w/chocolate frosting	1 piece	240	36	1	35	2	11
w/vanilla frosting	1 piece	240	38	Tr	38	2	9
CANDY	...	...	.	.	.	.	.
Almond Joy, 1.8 oz bar	1 bar	240	29	3	26	2	13
Baby Ruth, 2.1 oz bar	1 bar	280	40	1	39	3	13
Bit-O-Honey	6 pieces	150	32	Tr	32	Tr	3
Butterfinger, 2.1 oz bar	1 bar	280	44	1	43	3	11
Caramel	...	...	.	.	.	.	.
regular caramel, 0.3 oz	1 piece	40	8	0	8	Tr	Tr
regular caramel, 2.5 oz	1 pkg	270	55	0	55	3	6
chocolate caramel roll	1 piece	25	6	0	6	Tr	Tr
chocolate covered, with nuts	1 piece	70	9	Tr	9	1	3
Caramello, 1.6 oz bar	1 bar	210	29	Tr	29	3	10
Carob	1 oz	150	16	1	15	2	9
Charms Blow Pop	1	60	17	0	17	0	0
Chewing Gum-see Chewing Gum	...	...	.	.	.	.	.
Chocolate Bars	...	...	.	.	.	.	.
Hershey's Milk Chocolate, 1.5 oz	...	...	.	.	.	.	.
plain	1 bar	210	26	1	25	3	13
w/almonds	1 bar	210	21	2	19	4	14
Hershey's Special Dark, 1.5 oz	1 bar	180	25	3	22	2	12

	SERVING SIZE	CALORIES	TOTAL CARBS (g)	FIBER (g)	NET CARBS (g)	PROTEIN (g)	FAT (g)
Hershey's Extra Creamy Chocolate & Caramel, 1.25 oz	1 bar	180	22	Tr	22	2	9
Hershey's Miniatures, 1.5 oz	5 pc	210	25	2	23	3	13
Hershey's Mr. Goodbar, 1.75 oz	1 bar	250	26	2	24	5	17
(see "Chocolate for Baking" listed separately)	... ...	... ...	. .	. .	. .	. .	. .
Chocolate Coated Peanuts	10	210	20	2	18	5	13
Chocolate Coated Raisins	10	40	7	Tr	7	Tr	2
Chocolate Kiss, *Hershey's*	9 pc	230	24	1	23	3	13
Fifth Avenue bar, 2 oz	1 bar	270	35	2	33	5	13
Fruit Leather, pieces, 1 pkt	¾ oz	80	17	0	17	Tr	Tr
Fruit Leather, small roll	1 roll	50	12	0	12	Tr	Tr
Fudge, 1 piece	...	...	.	.	.	.	.
chocolate	¾ oz	90	16	Tr	16	Tr	2
chocolate w/nuts	¾ oz	100	14	Tr	14	Tr	4
chocolate w/ marshmallow	¾ oz	100	15	Tr	15	Tr	4
chocolate w/ marshmallow & nuts	¾ oz	100	14	Tr	14	Tr	4
peanut butter	¾ oz	80	16	Tr	16	Tr	1
vanilla	¾ oz	80	17	0	17	Tr	1
vanilla w/nuts	¾ oz	90	16	Tr	16	Tr	3
Goobers, 1.4 oz pkg	1	200	21	4	17	4	13
Gumdrops ¾" dia	5	80	21	0	21	0	0
Gummy Bears	10	90	22	0	22	0	0
Gummy Worms	10	290	73	Tr	73	0	0

	SERVING SIZE	CALORIES	TOTAL CARBS (g)	FIBER (g)	NET CARBS (g)	PROTEIN (g)	FAT (g)
Hard Candy	...	...	.	.	.	.	.
regular	2	45	12	0	12	0	Tr
butterscotch	2	40	10	0	10	0	Tr
sugar free	2	25	6	0	6	0	0
Jelly Beans, regular size	10	110	26	Tr	26	0	Tr
Jelly Beans, small pieces	10	40	10	0	10	0	Tr
Kit Kat bar, 1.5 oz	1 bar	220	27	Tr	27	3	11
Krackel bar, 1.5 oz	1 bar	210	26	Tr	26	3	11
M&M candy	...	...	.	.	.	.	.
plain	10	35	5	Tr	5	Tr	2
w/peanuts	10	100	12	1	12	2	5
w/almonds	10	170	20	2	18	3	9
Mars Almond bar, 1.75 oz	1 bar	230	31	1	30	4	12
Marshmallow, avg size (¼ oz)	1	25	6	0	6	Tr	Tr
Milky Way, regular size, 2 oz	1 bar	260	41	Tr	41	2	10
Milky Way, small, fun size	1 bar	80	12	Tr	12	Tr	3
Mounds, 1.9 oz bar	1 bar	260	31	2	29	2	14
Oh Henry!, 2 oz bar	1 bar	260	37	1	36	4	13
Oh Henry!, fun size bar	1 bar	120	17	Tr	17	2	6
Nestle Crunch bar, 1.55 oz	1 bar	220	30	Tr	30	2	11
Nestle Crunch bar, fun size	1 bar	50	7	Tr	7	Tr	3
Peanut Brittle	1 oz	140	20	Tr	20	2	5
Peppermint Pattie, 1.5 oz	1	170	35	Tr	35	Tr	3
Raisinets, 1.6 oz	1 pkg	190	31	1	30	2	8
Reese's Bites	16 pc	200	22	1	21	4	12

	SERVING SIZE	CALORIES	TOTAL CARBS (g)	FIBER (g)	NET CARBS (g)	PROTEIN (g)	FAT (g)
Reese's Fast Break	1 bar	280	36	2	34	5	13
Reese's Nutrageous, 1.92 oz	1 bar	280	29	2	27	6	17
Reese's Peanut Butter Cups	. . .	. . .	.	.	.	.	.
regular size cups	2 cups	230	25	2	23	5	14
miniature size cups	2 cups	70	8	Tr	8	1	4
Reese's Pieces, 1.6 oz pkg	1 pkg	230	28	1	27	6	11
Reese Sticks, 1.5 oz	1	220	23	1	22	4	13
Rolo caramels	7 pc	200	29	Tr	29	2	9
Skittles, original	10 pc	45	10	0	10	Tr	Tr
Skor toffee bar, 1.4 oz	1 bar	210	24	Tr	24	1	13
Snickers bar, regular size, 2 oz	1 bar	270	35	1	34	4	14
Snickers bar, small fun size	1 bar	70	9	Tr	9	1	4
Special Dark, miniature bar	1 bar	100	10	1	9	Tr	6
Starburst Fruit Chews, 2 oz	1 pkg	240	49	0	49	Tr	5
Three Musketeers, 2.1 oz	1 bar	260	46	Tr	46	2	8
Three Musketeers, fun size	1 bar	60	11	Tr	11	Tr	2
Toffee	1 oz	160	18	0	18	Tr	9
Tootsie Roll	6 pc	160	35	0	35	Tr	1
Twizzlers, Strawberry, 2.5 oz pkg	1 pkg	250	28	0	28	2	2
Whatchamacallit, 1.7 oz bar	1 bar	240	30	Tr	30	4	11
Cantaloupe	. . .	. . .	.	.	.	.	.
Fresh, medium size, 5" dia	1 melon	190	45	5	40	5	1

	SERVING SIZE	CALORIES	TOTAL CARBS (g)	FIBER (g)	NET CARBS (g)	PROTEIN (g)	FAT (g)
Fresh, wedge ⅛ melon	1 wedge	25	6	Tr	6	Tr	Tr
Fresh, cubed	1 cup	50	13	1	12	1	Tr
Fresh, balls	1 cup	60	14	2	12	2	Tr
Carambola (starfruit)	. . .	. . .	.	.	.	.	.
Fresh, 3 ⅝", whole	1	30	6	3	3	Tr	Tr
Fresh, sliced	1 cup	30	7	3	4	1	Tr
Caramels – see Candy	. . .	. . .	.	.	.	.	.
Carrot	. . .	. . .	.	.	.	.	.
Fresh, raw, whole, 7 ½" long	1	30	7	2	5	Tr	Tr
Fresh, raw, shredded	1 cup	45	11	3	8	1	Tr
Fresh, baby carrots, 3 oz	8–9 pc	30	7	3	4	Tr	Tr
Fresh, cooked, slices	1 cup	60	13	5	8	1	Tr
Frozen, cooked, slices	1 cup	50	11	5	7	Tr	Tr
Canned, drained, slices, cooked	1 cup	35	8	2	6	Tr	Tr
Cashew – see Nuts	. . .	. . .	.	.	.	.	.
Catsup, regular	1 Tbsp	15	4	0	4	Tr	Tr
Restaurant size packet	1 pkt	5	2	0	2	Tr	Tr
Cauliflower	. . .	. . .	.	.	.	.	.
Fresh, raw, flowerets	3	10	2	1	1	Tr	Tr
Fresh, raw, chopped or diced	1 cup	25	5	3	2	2	Tr
Fresh, flowerets, cooked	3	10	2	1	1	Tr	Tr
Fresh, chopped, cooked	1 cup	30	5	3	2	2	Tr
Frozen, chopped, cooked	1 cup	35	7	5	2	3	Tr
Caviar	1 Tbsp	40	Tr	0	Tr	4	3
Cayenne, dried spice	¼ tsp	0	Tr	Tr	Tr	Tr	Tr

	SERVING SIZE	CALORIES	TOTAL CARBS (g)	FIBER (g)	NET CARBS (g)	PROTEIN (g)	FAT (g)
Celery	...	...	.	.	.	.	.
Fresh, raw, stalk, 7 ½" long	1 stalk	5	1	Tr	1	Tr	Tr
Fresh, raw, diced	1 cup	15	3	2	1	Tr	Tr
Cooked, stalk 7 ½" long	2 stalks	15	3	1	2	Tr	Tr
Cooked, diced pieces	1 cup	25	6	2	4	1	Tr
Celery Seed	1 tsp	10	Tr	Tr	Tr	Tr	Tr
CEREAL	...	...	.	.	.	.	.
All-Bran	½ cup	80	23	9	14	4	2
Apple Jacks	1 cup	130	30	Tr	30	1	Tr
Cap'n Crunch	...	...	.	.	.	.	.
regular	¾ cup	110	23	Tr	23	1	2
Crunchberries	¾ cup	110	22	Tr	22	1	2
Peanut Butter Crunch	¾ cup	110	21	Tr	21	2	3
Cheerios Cereal, regular	1 cup	100	21	3	18	3	2
Apple Cinnamon Cheerios	¾ cup	120	25	1	24	2	2
Honey Nut Cheerios	¾ cup	110	22	2	20	3	2
Chex Cereal	...	...	.	.	.	.	.
Corn	1 cup	110	26	1	25	2	Tr
Frosted	¾ cup	110	27	0	27	1	Tr
Honey Nut	¾ cup	130	28	Tr	28	2	Tr
Multi Bran	¾ cup	150	40	6	34	3	1
Rice	1 cup	100	23	Tr	23	2	Tr
Wheat	¾ cup	170	38	5	33	5	Tr
Cinnamon Toast Crunch	¾ cup	130	25	1	24	2	3
Cocoa Krispies	¾ cup	120	27	Tr	27	2	Tr
Cocoa Puffs	¾ cup	110	23	1	22	Tr	1
Corn Flakes	1 cup	100	24	1	23	2	Tr
Kellogg's Corn Flakes	1 cup	100	24	Tr	24	2	Tr

	SERVING SIZE	CALORIES	TOTAL CARBS (g)	FIBER (g)	NET CARBS (g)	PROTEIN (g)	FAT (g)
Total Corn Flakes	1 cup	110	26	Tr	26	2	Tr
Corn Pops	1 cup	120	28	Tr	28	1	Tr
Cream of Rice, as prep	1 cup	130	28	Tr	28	2	Tr
Cream of Wheat, as prep	1 cup	150	32	1	31	4	Tr
Crispix	1 cup	110	26	Tr	26	2	Tr
Crispix Cinnamon Crunch	¾ cup	120	26	Tr	26	1	1
Froot Loops	1 cup	120	26	Tr	26	1	1
Froot Loops, reduced sugar	1¼ cup	130	28	1	27	2	1
Frosted Flakes	¾ cup	110	27	Tr	27	1	Tr
Frosted Flakes, reduced sugar	1 cup	120	28	Tr	28	2	Tr
Frosted Mini Wheats	. . .	. . .	.	.	.	.	.
regular size	5 biscuits	180	42	5	37	5	Tr
bite size	24 biscuits	200	48	6	42	6	Tr
Golden Grahams	¾ cup	120	26	1	25	1	1
Granola Cereal	. . .	. . .	.	.	.	.	.
homemade	1 cup	600	65	11	54	18	29
Kashi Mountain Medley	½ cup	220	37	6	31	6	7
Kashi Orchard Spice	½ cup	220	37	6	31	6	7
Kashi Summer Berry	½ cup	220	37	7	31	7	6
Kellogg's Low Fat w/ Raisins	½ cup	190	40	3	37	4	3
Kellogg's Low Fat w/ Raisins	⅔ cup	230	49	4	45	5	3
Nature Valley Low Fat Fruit	⅔ cup	210	44	3	41	4	3
Quaker Low Fat w/ Raisins	⅔ cup	220	45	3	42	4	3

	SERVING SIZE	CALORIES	TOTAL CARBS (g)	FIBER (g)	NET CARBS (g)	PROTEIN (g)	FAT (g)
Quaker Oats & Honey	½ cup	210	35	3	32	5	6
Quaker Sun Country Granola w/ almonds	½ cup	270	38	3	35	7	10
Kix Cereal, regular	1¼ cup	110	25	3	22	2	1
Kix Berry Berry	¾ cup	100	23	Tr	23	Tr	1
Life Cereal, regular	¾ cup	120	25	2	23	3	1
Life Cinnamon Cereal	¾ cup	120	25	2	23	3	1
Life Honey Graham	¾ cup	120	25	2	23	3	1
Lucky Charms	¾ cup	110	22	1	21	2	Tr
Lucky Charms, Chocolate	1 cup	120	26	1	25	1	1
Malt O Meal, as prep	1 cup	110	23	1	22	4	Tr
Malt O Meal, Chocolate, as prep	1 cup	120	25	1	24	3	Tr
Maltex, as prep	1 cup	190	39	2	37	6	1
Oatmeal, warm -see Oatmeal	. . .	. . .	.	.	.	.	.
Product 19	1 cup	100	25	1	24	2	Tr
Puffed Rice Cereal	1 cup	60	13	Tr	13	Tr	Tr
Puffed Rice, Quaker	1 cup	50	12	Tr	12	Tr	Tr
Puffed Wheat Cereal	1 cup	45	10	Tr	10	2	Tr
Raisin Bran Cereal	. . .	. . .	.	.	.	.	.
General Mills Raisin Nut Bran	¾ cup	200	42	5	37	4	4
General Mills Total Raisin Bran	1 cup	170	42	5	37	3	1
General Mills Wheaties Raisin Bran	1 cup	180	45	5	37	4	Tr
Kellogg's Raisin Bran	1 cup	190	46	7	39	5	1
Kellogg's Raisin Bran Crunch	1 cup	190	45	4	41	3	1

	SERVING SIZE	CALORIES	TOTAL CARBS (g)	FIBER (g)	NET CARBS (g)	PROTEIN (g)	FAT (g)
Kraft Post Raisin Bran	1 cup	190	45	7	38	6	2
Malt O Meal Raisin Bran	1 cup	210	45	8	37	5	1
Rice Crispies, *Kellogg's*	...	...	.	.	.	.	.
regular	1 ¼ cup	130	28	Tr	28	2	Tr
Berry Rice Crispies	1 cup	120	26	Tr	26	2	Tr
Frosted Rice Crispies	¾ cup	120	27	Tr	27	2	Tr
Rice Chex, General Mills	1 cup	100	23	Tr	23	2	Tr
Shredded wheat cereal,	...	...	.	.	.	.	.
Kellogg's Minatures	30 biscuits	100	24	4	20	3	Tr
large frosted biscuits	2 biscuits	160	36	6	30	5	1
Post Original Shredded Wheat Spoon Size	1 cup	170	41	6	35	5	Tr
Post Frosted Shredded Wheat	1 cup	180	44	5	39	4	Tr
Smacks Cereal	¾ cup	100	24	1	23	2	Tr
Special K	1 cup	120	22	Tr	22	7	Tr
Special K Low Carb	¾ cup	100	14	4	10	10	3
Total-see Raisin Bran	...	...	.	.	.	.	.
Total, Whole Grain	¾ cup	100	23	3	20	2	Tr
Trix Cereal	1 cup	130	28	1	27	1	2
Wheaties	¾ cup	100	22	3	19	3	Tr
Cereal Bar	...	...	.	.	.	.	.
Nutrigrain, Fruit filled	1 bar	140	27	Tr	27	2	3
Chalupa – see individual restaurant listings	...	...	.	.	.	.	.

	SERVING SIZE	CALORIES	TOTAL CARBS (g)	FIBER (g)	NET CARBS (g)	PROTEIN (g)	FAT (g)
CHEESE	...	...	.	.	.	.	.
American, pasteurized cheese	...	...	.	.	.	.	.
regular	1 oz	110	Tr	0	Tr	6	9
low fat	1 slice	40	Tr	0	Tr	5	2
fat free	1 slice	30	3	0	3	5	Tr
Blue cheese	1 oz	100	Tr	0	Tr	6	8
Camembert	1 oz	90	Tr	0	Tr	6	7
Cheddar cheese	...	...	.	.	.	.	.
regular, 1 slice	1 oz	110	Tr	0	Tr	7	9
1 inch cube	1	70	Tr	0	Tr	4	6
shredded	1 cup	460	2	0	2	28	38
lowfat	1 oz	50	Tr	0	Tr	7	2
Cheese food, pasteurized	1 oz	90	2	0	2	5	7
Cheese spread, cream cheese base	1 oz	80	Tr	0	Tr	2	8
Cheese spread, pasteurized	1 oz	80	3	0	3	5	6
Cheese Spread, Velveeta	1 oz	90	3	0	3	5	6
Colby cheese	1 oz	110	Tr	0	Tr	7	9
Colby cheese, low fat	1 oz	50	Tr	0	Tr	7	2
Cottage cheese	...	...	.	.	.	.	.
regular, creamed, 4% fat	...	...	.	.	.	.	.
large curd	1 cup	210	7	0	7	23	9
small curd	1 cup	220	8	0	8	25	10
with fruit	1 cup	220	10	Tr	10	24	9
lowfat, 2% fat	1 cup	190	8	0	8	27	6
lowfat, 1% fat	1 cup	160	6	0	6	28	2
lowfat, 1% fat w/ vegetables	1 cup	150	7	0	7	25	2
fat free	1 cup	100	10	0	10	15	Tr

	SERVING SIZE	CALORIES	TOTAL CARBS (g)	FIBER (g)	NET CARBS (g)	PROTEIN (g)	FAT (g)
dry curd, uncreamed, nonfat	1 cup	100	10	0	10	15	Tr
Cream cheese	...	...	.	.	.	.	.
regular cream	1 oz	100	1	0	1	2	10
regular cream	1 Tbsp	50	Tr	0	Tr	Tr	5
regular cream, whipped	1 Tbsp	35	Tr	0	Tr	Tr	3
lowfat/light	1 Tbsp	30	1	0	1	1	2
lowfat, whipped	1 Tbsp	20	Tr	0	Tr	Tr	2
fat free	1 oz	30	2	0	2	4	Tr
Feta cheese	1 oz	80	1	0	1	4	6
Feta cheese, crumbled	1 cup	400	6	0	6	21	32
Fontina cheese	1 oz	110	Tr	0	Tr	7	9
Fontina cheese, shredded	1 cup	420	2	0	2	28	34
Goat cheese, soft	1 oz	80	Tr	0	Tr	5	6
Goat cheese, semisoft	1 oz	100	Tr	0	Tr	6	9
Goat cheese, hard	1 oz	130	Tr	0	Tr	9	10
Monterey cheese	1 oz	110	Tr	0	Tr	7	9
Monterey cheese, shredded	1 cup	420	Tr	0	Tr	28	34
Monterey cheese, low fat	1 oz	90	Tr	0	Tr	8	6
Monterey cheese, low fat, shredded	1 cup	350	Tr	0	Tr	32	24
Mozzarella cheese, whole milk	...	...	.	.	.	.	.
regular, 1 slice	1 oz	90	Tr	0	Tr	6	6
shredded	1 cup	340	3	0	3	25	25
Mozzarella cheese, part skim milk	1 oz	70	Tr	0	Tr	7	5
Mozzarella cheese, fat free, shredded	1 cup	170	4	2	2	36	0

	SERVING SIZE	CALORIES	TOTAL CARBS (g)	FIBER (g)	NET CARBS (g)	PROTEIN (g)	FAT (g)
Muenster cheese	...	...	.	.	.	.	.
sliced	1 oz	100	Tr	0	Tr	7	9
shredded	1 cup	420	1	0	1	27	34
Muenster cheese, low fat, slice	1 oz	80	Tr	0	Tr	7	5
Neufchatel cheese	1 oz	70	1	0	1	3	7
Parmesan cheese	...	...	.	.	.	.	.
grated	1 cup	430	4	0	4	39	29
grated	1 Tbsp	20	Tr	0	Tr	2	1
Provolone cheese	1 oz	100	Tr	0	Tr	7	8
Provolone cheese, reduced fat	1 oz	80	Tr	0	Tr	7	5
Ricotta cheese	...	...	.	.	.	.	.
regular	1 cup	430	8	0	8	28	32
part skim	1 cup	340	13	0	13	28	20
Romano cheese, grated	1 oz	110	1	0	1	9	8
Roquefort, sheep's milk	1 oz	110	Tr	0	Tr	6	9
Swiss cheese	...	...	.	.	.	.	.
regular, 1 slice	1 oz	110	2	0	2	8	8
regular, shredded	1 cup	410	6	0	6	29	30
low fat, 1 slice	1 oz	50	Tr	0	Tr	8	1
low fat, shredded	1 oz	190	4	0	4	31	6
Cheese Puffs or Twists	1 oz	160	15	Tr	15	2	10
Cheez Whiz	2 Tbsp	90	3	Tr	3	4	7
Cheez Whiz Light	2 Tbsp	80	6	Tr	6	6	3
Cherries	...	...	.	.	.	.	.
Fresh, sweet	10	50	13	2	11	Tr	Tr
Sweet, canned, water packed	1 cup	110	29	4	25	2	Tr
Sour, canned, water pack	1 cup	90	22	3	19	2	Tr

	SERVING SIZE	CALORIES	TOTAL CARBS (g)	FIBER (g)	NET CARBS (g)	PROTEIN (g)	FAT (g)
Sour, frozen, unsweetened	1 cup	70	17	3	14	1	Tr
Cherry Pie Filling, canned	3 oz	100	24	Tr	24	Tr	Tr
Chestnut – see Nuts	. . .	. . .	.	.	.	.	.
Chewing Gum	. . .	. . .	.	.	.	.	.
Chicklets	10	40	11	Tr	11	0	Tr
Stick	1	7	2	Tr	2	0	Tr
Block	1	20	5	Tr	5	0	Tr
Sugarless	1 piece	5	2	0	2	0	Tr
Wrigley's, regular	1 stick	10	2	0	2	0	0
Wrigley's Eclipse	2 pieces	5	2	0	2	0	0
Wrigley's Extra, sugarfree	1 stick	5	2	0	2	0	0
Bubble Yum, all regular flavors	1	25	6	0	6	0	0
Dentyne Ice, all flavors	2	5	2	0	2	0	0
Ice Breakers	1	10	2	0	2	0	0
Trident, all flavors, 1" sticks	1 stick	5	1	0	1	0	0
Chex Mix, 1 oz	⅔ cup	120	21	1	20	3	3
CHICKEN	. . .	. . .	.	.	.	.	.
Giblets, simmered, chopped	1 cup	230	Tr	0	Tr	39	7
Fried Chicken, batter dipped	. . .	. . .	.	.	.	.	.
½ Breast, bone removed	5 oz	360	13	Tr	13	35	19
Drumstick, avg size	1	190	6	Tr	6	16	11
Thigh, avg size	1	240	8	Tr	8	19	14
Wing, avg size	1	160	5	Tr	5	10	11
Fried Chicken, boneless pieces, breaded	6 pieces	290	16	Tr	16	15	18

	SERVING SIZE	CALORIES	TOTAL CARBS (g)	FIBER (g)	NET CARBS (g)	PROTEIN (g)	FAT (g)
Liver of chicken, simmered	3 oz	140	Tr	0	Tr	21	6
Neck, simmered	1	90	0	0	0	8	7
Roasted Chicken	...	...	.	.	.	.	.
½ Breast, bone removed	3.5 oz	190	0	0	0	29	8
Drumstick, avg size	1	110	0	0	0	14	6
Thigh, avg size	1	150	0	0	0	16	10
Wing, avg size	1	100	0	0	0	9	7
White meat skinless, chopped	1 cup	210	0	0	0	38	6
Dark meat skinless, chopped	1 cup	250	0	0	0	33	13
Light & dark skinless, chopped	1 cup	230	0	0	0	35	9
Canned, boneless	5 oz	230	0	0	0	32	10
Stewed Chicken	...	...	.	.	.	.	.
Breast, skinless, chopped	1 cup	210	0	0	0	41	4
Dark meat skinless, chopped	1 cup	270	0	0	0	36	13
Light & dark meat, skinless, chopped	1 cup	250	0	0	0	38	10
Drumstick, skinless	1	80	0	0	0	13	3
Thigh, skinless	1	110	0	0	0	14	5
(Other Chicken Products, see:	...	...	.	.	.	.	.
Bologna, Hot Dog, Salami,	...	...	.	.	.	.	.
Sausage & specific entrées)	...	...	.	.	.	.	.
Chicken Nuggets	...	...	.	.	.	.	.
Frozen, cooked	3 oz	250	12	2	10	13	17

	SERVING SIZE	CALORIES	TOTAL CARBS (g)	FIBER (g)	NET CARBS (g)	PROTEIN (g)	FAT (g)
Chicken Roll, light meat	2 oz	60	3	0	3	10	2
Chickpeas, cooked	½ cup	130	23	6	17	7	2
Chili Powder	1 tsp	10	1	Tr	1	Tr	Tr
Chili w/Beans, *Hormel, canned*	1 cup	190	18	3	15	17	7
Chili Con Carne w/Beans, canned	1 cup	300	28	10	18	17	13
Chimichanga – see individual restaurant listings	. . .	. . .	.	.	.	.	.
Chips – see Corn Chips, Potato	. . .	. . .	.	.	.	.	.
Chips & other specific listings	. . .	. . .	.	.	.	.	.
Chives, raw, chopped	1 Tbsp	0	Tr	Tr	Tr	Tr	Tr
Chives, freeze-dried	1 Tbsp	0	Tr	Tr	Tr	Tr	Tr
Chocolate for Baking (Also see	. . .	. . .	.	.	.	.	.
"Candy" for other chocolates)	. . .	. . .	.	.	.	.	.
Mexican baking chocolate	1 sq	90	16	Tr	16	Tr	3
Nestlé Milk Chocolate Morsels	1 Tbsp	70	9	0	9	Tr	4
Nestlè Semi-Sweet Chocolate Morsels	1 Tbsp	70	9	Tr	9	Tr	4
Nestlè Premier White Chocolate Morsels	1 Tbsp	70	9	0	9	0	4
Unsweetened for baking, solid	1 sq	150	9	5	4	4	15
Unsweetened, liquid	1 oz	130	10	5	5	3	14
Cilantro, raw	¼ cup	0	Tr	Tr	Tr	Tr	Tr
Cilantro, dried	1 tsp	0	Tr	Tr	Tr	Tr	Tr

	SERVING SIZE	CALORIES	TOTAL CARBS (g)	FIBER (g)	NET CARBS (g)	PROTEIN (g)	FAT (g)
Cinnamon	1 tsp	5	2	1	1	Tr	Tr
Cinnamon Sweet Roll	...	...	.	.	.	.	.
w/ raisins & glaze, 2¾"	1	220	31	1	30	4	10
Cinnamon Roll w/icing, *Pillsbury*	1	150	23	Tr	23	2	5
Clam Chowder – see Soup	...	...	.	.	.	.	.
Clams – see Fish/Seafood	...	...	.	.	.	.	.
Cloves, ground	1 tsp	5	1	Tr	1	Tr	Tr
Cocoa, unsweetened	1 Tbsp	10	3	2	1	1	Tr
powder	1 cup	200	50	29	21	17	12
Coconut	...	...	.	.	.	.	.
Fresh piece, 2" × 2" × ½"	1 piece	160	7	4	3	2	15
Fresh, shredded, not packed	1 cup	280	12	7	5	3	27
Dried, sweetened, shredded	1 cup	460	44	4	40	3	33
Dried, unsweetened	1 oz	190	7	5	2	2	18
Coconut cream, canned, sweetened	1 Tbsp	70	10	0	10	Tr	3
Coconut milk, canned	1 cup	450	6	0	6	5	48
Coleslaw	½ cup	45	8	Tr	8	Tr	2
Collards	...	...	.	.	.	.	.
Fresh, chopped, cooked	1 cup	50	9	5	4	4	Tr
Frozen, chopped, cooked	1 cup	60	12	5	7	5	Tr
Condiments, see Sauce,	...	...	.	.	.	.	.
or see specific listing	...	...	.	.	.	.	.
COOKIES 2 ¼" dia unless noted	...	...	.	.	.	.	.

	SERVING SIZE	CALORIES	TOTAL CARBS (g)	FIBER (g)	NET CARBS (g)	PROTEIN (g)	FAT (g)
Animal Crackers, 1" dia, sm box	2 oz	250	42	Tr	42	4	8
Butter Cookie	1	25	4	0	4	Tr	Tr
Chocolate Chip, regular	1	80	9	Tr	9	Tr	5
Chocolate Chip, reduced fat	1	45	7	Tr	7	Tr	2
Coconut cookie, 2"	1	100	17	Tr	17	Tr	3
Fig Bar	1	60	11	Tr	11	Tr	1
Molasses cookie	1	70	11	Tr	11	Tr	2
Oatmeal w/ raisins, 2⅝"	1	70	10	Tr	10	Tr	2
Oatmeal, plain, 2⅝"	1	70	10	Tr	10	1	3
Peanut Butter, plain, 3"	1	100	12	Tr	12	2	5
Pecan Shortbread cookie, 2"	1	80	8	Tr	8	Tr	5
Sandwich cookie, w/ filling,	...	...	.	.	.	.	.
1 ½" dia, round,	...	...	.	.	.	.	.
chocolate w/ creme filling	1	50	8	Tr	8	Tr	2
chocolate w/ creme filling, chocolate coated	1	80	11	Tr	11	Tr	5
chocolate w/ extra creme filling	1	70	9	Tr	9	Tr	3
peanut butter sandwich	1	70	9	Tr	9	1	3
sugar wafer w/ creme filling, small	1	20	3	0	3	Tr	Tr
sugar wafer w/ creme filling, large	1	45	6	Tr	6	Tr	2
vanilla w/ creme filling	1	50	7	Tr	7	Tr	2

	SERVING SIZE	CALORIES	TOTAL CARBS (g)	FIBER (g)	NET CARBS (g)	PROTEIN (g)	FAT (g)
vanilla w/ creme filling, oval	1	70	11	Tr	11	Tr	3
Shortbread cookie, plain, 1 ⅝" square	1	40	5	Tr	5	Tr	2
Sugar Cookie, regular	1	70	10	Tr	10	Tr	3
Wafer, chocolate	1	25	4	Tr	4	Tr	Tr
Wafer, vanilla	1	30	4	Tr	4	Tr	1
Wafer, vanilla, low fat	1	20	3	Tr	3	Tr	Tr
Cooking Spray, nonstick	. . .	. . .	.	.	.	.	.
⅓ second spray	1 spray	0	Tr	0	Tr	0	Tr
Corn	. . .	. . .	.	.	.	.	.
Sweet White or Yellow, 7" cob, cooked	1 ear	110	26	3	23	3	1
Canned, drained solids	½ cup	70	15	2	13	2	Tr
Canned, cream style kernels	½ cup	90	23	2	21	2	Tr
Frozen kernels, cooked	½ cup	70	16	2	14	2	Tr
Corn Cake, butter flavor	1	40	8	Tr	8	Tr	Tr
(also see Rice Cake)	. . .	. . .	.	.	.	.	.
Corn Chips	. . .	. . .	.	.	.	.	.
Regular	1 oz	150	18	2	16	2	8
Barbecue flavor	1 oz	150	16	2	14	2	9
Tortilla type	. . .	. . .	.	.	.	.	.
yellow corn	1 oz	140	19	1	18	2	6
white corn	1 oz	140	19	2	17	2	7
low fat	1 oz	120	23	2	21	3	2
nacho cheese	1 oz	150	18	1	17	2	7

	SERVING SIZE	CALORIES	TOTAL CARBS (g)	FIBER (g)	NET CARBS (g)	PROTEIN (g)	FAT (g)
nacho flavor, reduced fat	1 oz	130	20	1	19	3	4
ranch flavor	1 oz	140	18	1	17	2	7
taco flavor	1 oz	140	18	2	16	2	7
Corn Grits (hominy) – see Grits	...	...	.	.	.	.	.
Corn Syrup, light	1 Tbsp	60	17	0	17	0	Tr
dark	1 Tbsp	60	16	0	16	0	0
Cornbread, 2× 3″	1 piece	190	29	1	28	4	6
Corned Beef	3 oz	210	0	0	0	23	13
Corned Beef Hash, canned	...	...	.	.	.	.	.
Hormel	1 cup	390	22	3	19	21	24
Cornish Hen, roasted	½ bird	340	0	0	0	29	24
Cornmeal, yellow or white, dry form	...	...	.	.	.	.	.
Whole grain	1 cup	440	94	9	85	10	4
Self rising	1 cup	490	103	10	93	12	2
Cornstarch	1 Tbsp	30	7	Tr	7	Tr	Tr
Cottage cheese – see Cheese	...	...	.	.	.	.	.
Crab – see Fish	...	...	.	.	.	.	.
Crabcake	1	160	5	Tr	5	11	10
Cracker Jacks	½ cup	120	23	1	22	2	2
CRACKERS	...	...	.	.	.	.	.
Cheese crackers, 1″ squares	10	50	6	Tr	6	1	3
Club crackers, *Keebler Club*	4	70	9	Tr	9	Tr	3
Graham crackers, 2 ½″ sq	3	90	16	Tr	16	2	2
Matzo, plain, 6″ square	1	110	23	Tr	23	3	Tr

	SERVING SIZE	CALORIES	TOTAL CARBS (g)	FIBER (g)	NET CARBS (g)	PROTEIN (g)	FAT (g)
Melba toast, plain	4	45	9	Tr	9	2	Tr
Oyster crackers	25	110	19	Tr	19	2	2
Ritz Bitz w/peanut butter, 1.25 oz bag	1	170	20	1	19	4	10
Ritz crackers, regular	5	80	10	Tr	10	1	4
Ritz crackers, reduced fat	5	70	11	0	11	1	2
Rye crispbread	...	...	.	.	.	.	.
Rye Krisp wafer	1	90	21	4	17	2	Tr
Wasa Rye	1	35	8	2	6	Tr	Tr
Saltine crackers	5	60	11	Tr	11	1	1
Sandwich crackers, 1 ½" dia,	...	...	.	.	.	.	.
cheese filled	2	60	8	Tr	8	1	3
cheese cracker, peanut butter filled	2	60	7	Tr	7	2	3
peanut butter filled	2	70	8	Tr	8	2	3
Snack crackers, round, 2" dia	5	80	10	Tr	10	1	4
Sociables	7	70	9	0	9	1	4
Town House crackers	5	80	10	Tr	10	Tr	5
Whole wheat, thin squares	8	80	10	Tr	10	1	3
Cranberries	...	.	.	.	.	.	.
Fresh, raw, unsweetened	½ cup	25	6	2	4	Tr	Tr
Dried, sweetened	¼ cup	90	25	2	23	Tr	Tr
Cranberry-orange Relish	2 Tbsp	60	16	0	16	Tr	Tr
Cranberry Sauce, sweet, canned	1 slice	90	22	Tr	22	Tr	Tr

	SERVING SIZE	CALORIES	TOTAL CARBS (g)	FIBER (g)	NET CARBS (g)	PROTEIN (g)	FAT (g)
Cream Cheese – see Cheese	...	...	.	.	.	.	.
Cream of Tartar	1 tsp	10	2	0	2	0	0
Cream of Wheat Cereal, as prep	1 cup	130	28	1	27	4	Tr
Cream of Wheat Cereal, instant, as prep	1 cup	150	32	1	31	4	Tr
Cream Puff, 2″ × 3½″	1	290	27	Tr	27	7	18
Cream, Whipped Topping	.	.	.	.	.	.	.
Light, whipped	2 cups	700	7	0	7	5	74
Light, whipped	2 Tbsp	45	Tr	0	Tr	Tr	5
Heavy, whipped	2 cups	820	7	0	7	5	88
Heavy, whipped	2 Tbsp	50	Tr	0	Tr	Tr	6
Pressurized in can	1 Tbsp	10	Tr	0	Tr	Tr	Tr
Creamer-see Beverages, Creamer	...	...	.	.	.	.	.
Croissant, butter flavor, 4″	1	230	26	2	24	5	12
Croissant w/Egg, Bacon, Cheese – see Breakfast Sandwich	...	...	.	.	.	.	.
Croutons, plain	½ cup	60	11	Tr	11	2	Tr
Croutons, seasoned	½ cup	90	13	1	12	2	4
Cucumber	...	...	.	.	.	.	.
Fresh, peeled, whole, 8¼″ long	1	35	6	2	4	2	Tr
Fresh, peeled, sliced	1 cup	15	3	Tr	3	Tr	Tr
Fresh, unpeeled, whole 8¼″ long	1	45	11	2	9	2	Tr
Fresh, unpeeled, sliced	1 cup	15	4	Tr	4	Tr	Tr

	SERVING SIZE	CALORIES	TOTAL CARBS (g)	FIBER (g)	NET CARBS (g)	PROTEIN (g)	FAT (g)
Cucumber Salad, mayo dressing	¾ cup	120	9	2	7	2	10
Curry Powder	1 tsp	5	1	Tr	1	Tr	Tr
Custard, egg	. . .	. . .	.	.	.	.	.
Vanilla	½ cup	150	15	0	15	7	7
Caramel (flan)	½ cup	220	35	0	35	7	6
Dandelion Greens, chopped, cooked	1 cup	35	7	3	4	2	Tr
Danish Pastry, approx 4" dia	. . .	. . .	.	.	.	.	.
Cheese	1	270	26	Tr	26	6	16
Cinnamon	1	260	29	Tr	29	5	15
Fruit filled	1	260	34	1	33	4	13
Lemon	1	260	34	1	33	4	13
Nut	1	280	30	1	29	5	16
Dates, Medjool, pitted	1	70	18	2	16	Tr	Tr
Dates, Deglet Noor, pitted	. . .	. . .	.	.	.	.	.
Whole	1	20	5	Tr	5	Tr	Tr
Chopped	1 cup	420	110	11	99	4	Tr
Dessert – see Ice Cream, Frozen	. . .	. . .	.	.	.	.	.
Dessert, or specific listing	. . .	. . .	.	.	.	.	.
Dessert Filling – see specific	. . .	. . .	.	.	.	.	.
listing	. . .	. . .	.	.	.	.	.
Dessert Topping – see Topping	. . .	. . .	.	.	.	.	.
Dill Seed	1 tsp	5	1	Tr	1	Tr	Tr
Dill Weed	. . .	. . .	.	.	.	.	.
Raw, sprigs	5	0	Tr	0	Tr	Tr	Tr
Dried	1 tsp	0	Tr	Tr	Tr	Tr	Tr

	SERVING SIZE	CALORIES	TOTAL CARBS (g)	FIBER (g)	NET CARBS (g)	PROTEIN (g)	FAT (g)
Doughnut	...	...	.	.	.	.	.
Cake Doughnuts	...	...	.	.	.	.	.
Regular ring type, approx 3" dia	...	...	.	.	.	.	.
Plain	1	230	25	Tr	25	3	13
Sugared or glazed	1	190	23	Tr	23	2	10
Chocolate, sugared or glazed	1	180	24	Tr	24	2	8
Chocolate frosting	1	190	22	Tr	22	2	11
French cruller, glazed	1	170	24	Tr	24	1	8
Yeast Doughnuts	...	...	...	.	.	.	.
Regular ring type, approz 3" dia	...	...	...	.	.	.	.
Glazed	1	240	27	Tr	27	4	14
Filled doughnuts	...	...	.	.	.	.	.
Creme filled	1	310	26	Tr	26	5	21
Jelly filled	1	290	33	Tr	33	5	16
Dressing – see Salad Dressing	...	...	.	.	.	.	.
Dried Fruit – see specific	...	...	.	.	.	.	.
listings, and Trail Mix	...	...	.	.	.	.	.
Duck, roasted	...	.	.	.	.	.	.
½ Duck, meat only	½ duck	440	0	0	0	52	25
meat only, chopped	1 cup	280	0	0	0	33	16
Èclair, 5" × 2"	1	260	24	Tr	24	6	16
EGG	...	...	.	.	.	.	.
Raw Eggs	...	...	.	.	.	.	.
1 medium whole egg	1	60	Tr	0	Tr	6	4
1 large whole egg	1	70	Tr	0	Tr	6	5
1 extra large whole egg	1	80	Tr	0	Tr	7	6

	SERVING SIZE	CALORIES	TOTAL CARBS (g)	FIBER (g)	NET CARBS (g)	PROTEIN (g)	FAT (g)
1 yolk only, large	1	50	Tr	0	Tr	3	5
1 white only, large	1	15	Tr	0	Tr	4	Tr
Prepared Eggs (1 Lg egg/svg)	...	...	.	.	.	.	.
hard boiled, whole	1	80	Tr	0	Tr	6	5
hard boiled, chopped	1 cup	210	2	0	2	17	14
omelet	1	100	Tr	0	Tr	7	7
fried	1	90	Tr	0	Tr	6	7
poached	1	70	Tr	0	Tr	6	5
scrambled	1	100	1	0	1	7	8
Egg Substitute or imitation	...	...	.	.	.	.	.
liquid	1.5 fl oz	40	Tr	0	Tr	6	2
frozen	¼ cup	100	2	0	2	7	7
powdered	⅓ oz	45	2	0	2	6	1
Eggplant	...	...	.	.	.	.	.
Cubed, cooked	1 cup	35	9	3	6	Tr	Tr
Eggplant Parmagiana	½ cup	265	26	3	23	6	16
Eggroll	...	...	.	.	.	.	.
chicken	1	160	23	2	21	8	4
pork	1	190	25	2	23	9	6
vegetable	1	150	25	2	23	5	4
Enchilada – see frozen dinner/ individual restaurant listings	...	...	.	.	.	.	.
Enchirito – see individual restaurant listings	...	...	.	.	.	.	.
Endive	...	...	.	.	.	.	.
head	1	90	17	16	1	6	1
raw, chopped	1 cup	10	2	2	0	Tr	Tr

	SERVING SIZE	CALORIES	TOTAL CARBS (g)	FIBER (g)	NET CARBS (g)	PROTEIN (g)	FAT (g)
Energy Bar, low carb	...	...	·	·	·	·	·
Atkins Advantage Chocolate Chip Granola Bar	1 bar	200	18	6	12	17	8
Atkins Advantage S'mores	1 bar	220	27	12	15	17	9
English Muffin-see BREAD	...	...	·	·	·	·	·
English Muffin w/ Egg, Cheese, & Canadian Bacon-see Breakfast Sandwich	...	...	·	·	·	·	·
Equal sweetener	1 pkt	0	Tr	0	Tr	Tr	0
Fig	...	...	·	·	·	·	·
dried	1	20	5	Tr	5	Tr	Tr
fresh, medium	1	35	10	2	8	Tr	Tr
FISH/SEAFOOD	...	...	·	·	·	·	·
Abalone, fried	3 oz	160	9	0	9	17	6
Anchovy, canned in oil	5	40	0	0	0	6	2
Bass	...	...	·	·	·	·	·
freshwater, baked	3 oz	120	0	0	0	21	4
striped, baked	3 oz	110	0	0	0	19	3
sea bass, baked	3 oz	110	0	0	0	20	2
Bluefish, baked	3 oz	140	0	0	0	22	5
Catfish	...	...	·	·	·	·	·
farmed, baked	3 oz	130	0	0	0	16	7
breaded, fried	3 oz	200	7	Tr	7	15	11
wild, baked	3 oz	90	0	0	0	16	2
Caviar, black or red	1 Tbsp	40	Tr	0	Tr	4	3
Clams	...	...	·	·	·	·	·
breaded, fried	¾ cup	450	39	Tr	39	13	26
canned, drained	3 oz	130	4	0	4	22	2

	SERVING SIZE	CALORIES	TOTAL CARBS (g)	FIBER (g)	NET CARBS (g)	PROTEIN (g)	FAT (g)
canned, drained	1 cup	240	8	0	8	41	3
raw	3 oz	60	2	0	2	11	Tr
raw	1 med	10	Tr	0	Tr	2	Tr
steamed	3 oz	130	4	0	4	22	2
Cod, baked or broiled	3 oz	90	0	0	0	20	Tr
Crab, Alaska king	. . .	. . .	.	.	.	.	.
steamed	3 oz	80	0	0	0	17	1
steamed	1 leg	130	0	0	0	26	2
Crab, blue	. . .	. . .	.	.	.	.	.
steamed	3 oz	90	0	0	0	17	2
canned	3 oz	80	0	0	0	17	1
Crab, Dungeness, steamed	3 oz	90	Tr	0	Tr	19	1
Crab, imitation crab meat	3 oz	80	13	Tr	13	7	Tr
Crab cake	1	160	5	Tr	5	11	10
Fish fillet, breaded, fried	3 oz	200	14	Tr	14	13	11
Fish stick, breaded, fried, 4" × 1"	1	70	6	Tr	6	3	4
Flounder	. . .	. . .	.	.	.	.	.
baked or broiled	3 oz	100	0	0	0	21	1
Grouper, baked or broiled	3 oz	100	0	0	0	21	1
Haddock	. . .	. . .	.	.	.	.	.
baked or broiled	3 oz	100	0	0	0	21	Tr
smoked	3 oz	100	0	0	0	22	Tr
Halibut	. . .	. . .	.	.	.	.	.
baked or broiled	3 oz	120	0	0	0	23	3
Herring, Atlantic	. . .	. . .	.	.	.	.	.
baked or broiled	3 oz	170	0	0	0	20	10
kippered, med fillet	1	90	0	0	0	10	5

	SERVING SIZE	CALORIES	TOTAL CARBS (g)	FIBER (g)	NET CARBS (g)	PROTEIN (g)	FAT (g)
pickled	1 oz	70	3	0	3	4	5
Herring, Pacific	...	...	.	.	.	.	.
baked or broiled	3 oz	210	0	0	0	18	15
Lobster, steamed	3 oz	80	1	0	1	17	Tr
Mackerel	...	...	.	.	.	.	.
Atlantic, baked or broiled	3 oz	220	0	0	0	20	15
king, baked or broiled	3 oz	110	0	0	0	22	2
Pacific and jack, baked or broiled	3 oz	170	0	0	0	22	9
jack, canned	1 cup	300	0	0	0	44	12
Spanish, baked or broiled	3 oz	130	0	0	0	20	5
salted	1 piece	240	0	0	0	15	10
Monkfish, baked or broiled	3 oz	80	0	0	0	16	2
Mussels, steamed	3 oz	150	6	0	6	20	4
Orange roughy, baked or broiled	3 oz	90	0	0	0	19	Tr
Oyster, Eastern	...	...	.	.	.	.	.
canned	3 oz	60	3	0	3	6	2
farmed, raw meat	6 med	50	5	0	5	4	1
farmed, baked or broiled	6 med	50	4	0	4	4	1
wild, raw meat	6 med	60	3	0	3	6	2
wild, baked or broiled	6 med	40	3	0	3	5	1
wild, steamed	6 med	60	3	0	3	6	2
breaded, fried	3 oz	170	10	1	9	8	11
Oyster, Pacific	...	...	.	.	.	.	.
raw	6 med	240	15	0	15	28	7
steamed	6 med	250	15	0	15	28	7

	SERVING SIZE	CALORIES	TOTAL CARBS (g)	FIBER (g)	NET CARBS (g)	PROTEIN (g)	FAT (g)
Perch, baked or broiled	3 oz	100	0	0	0	20	2
Pike, baked or broiled	3 oz	100	0	0	0	21	Tr
Pollock, baked or broiled	3 oz	100	0	0	0	21	1
Pompano, baked or broiled	3 oz	180	0	0	0	20	10
Rockfish, baked or broiled	3 oz	100	0	0	0	20	2
Salmon, Atlantic	. . .	. . .	.	.	.	.	.
farmed, baked or broiled	3 oz	180	0	0	0	19	11
wild, baked or broiled	3 oz	160	0	0	0	22	7
Salmon, coho	. . .	. . .	.	.	.	.	.
farmed, baked or broiled	3 oz	150	0	0	0	21	7
wild, baked or broiled	3 oz	120	0	0	0	20	4
Salmon, pink, canned	3 oz	120	0	0	0	20	4
Salmon, chinook, smoked, (lox)	3 oz	100	0	0	0	16	4
Sardines, canned in oil, drained	2	50	0	0	0	6	3
Scallop	. . .	. . .	.	.	.	.	.
breaded, fried	6 large	200	9	Tr	9	17	10
bay or sea, steamed	3 oz	100	0	0	0	20	1
Shark	. . .	. . .	.	.	.	.	.
battered and fried	3 oz	190	5	0	5	16	12
Shrimp	. . .	. . .	.	.	.	.	.

	SERVING SIZE	CALORIES	TOTAL CARBS (g)	FIBER (g)	NET CARBS (g)	PROTEIN (g)	FAT (g)
breaded, fried	4 large	70	3	Tr	3	6	4
breaded, fried	3 oz	210	10	Tr	10	18	10
canned, drained	3 oz	90	0	0	0	17	1
steamed	3 oz	80	0	0	0	18	Tr
Snapper, baked or broiled	3 oz	110	0	0	0	22	2
Sole	. . .	. . .	.	.	.	.	.
baked or broiled	3 oz	100	0	0	0	21	1
Squid, fried	3 oz	150	7	0	7	15	6
Swordfish, baked or broiled	3 oz	130	0	0	0	22	4
Trout, baked or broiled	3 oz	160	0	0	0	23	7
Trout, rainbow	. . .	. . .	.	.	.	.	.
farmed, baked or broiled	3 oz	140	0	0	0	21	6
wild, baked or broiled	3 oz	130	0	0	0	20	5
Tuna	. . .	. . .	.	.	.	.	.
bluefin, baked or broiled	3 oz	160	0	0	0	25	5
skipjack, baked or broiled	3 oz	110	0	0	0	24	1
yellowfin	3 oz	120	0	0	0	26	1
canned in oil, drained	3 oz	160	0	0	0	23	7
canned in water, chunk light	3 oz	100	0	0	0	22	Tr
canned in water, solid white	3 oz	110	0	0	0	20	3
tuna salad, oil packed, w/mayo	½ cup	190	10	0	10	16	10

	SERVING SIZE	CALORIES	TOTAL CARBS (g)	FIBER (g)	NET CARBS (g)	PROTEIN (g)	FAT (g)
tuna salad, water packed, w/	...	...	·	·	·	·	·
Whiting, baked or broiled	3 oz	100	0	0	0	20	1
Fish Sandwich, w/ tartar sauce	1	430	41	Tr	41	17	23
w/ tartar sauce & cheese	1	520	48	Tr	48	21	29
Flank Steak – see Beef	...	...	·	·	·	·	·
Flour, unsifted	...	...	·	·	·	·	·
All purpose flour, white	1 cup	460	95	3	92	13	1
Bread flour	1 cup	500	99	3	96	16	2
Buckwheat flour, whole groat	1 cup	400	85	12	73	15	4
Cake or pastry flour	1 cup	500	107	2	105	11	1
Carob flour	1 cup	230	92	41	51	5	Tr
Self-rising flour, white	1 cup	440	93	3	90	12	1
Rice flour	1 cup	580	127	4	123	9	2
Whole wheat flour	1 cup	410	87	15	72	16	2
Frankfurter – see Hot Dog	...	...	·	·	·	·	·
Freezer Pop – see Frozen Dessert	...	...	·	·	·	·	·
French Fries	...	...	·	·	·	·	·
Frozen, heated,	...	...	·	·	·	·	·
thin, shoestring strips	10	40	7	Tr	7	Tr	1
regular or crinkle cut	10	120	19	2	17	2	4
steak fries	10	200	36	4	32	3	5
French Toast	2 slices	250	38	1	37	9	7

	SERVING SIZE	CALORIES	TOTAL CARBS (g)	FIBER (g)	NET CARBS (g)	PROTEIN (g)	FAT (g)
Fried Chicken – see Chicken	...	...	.	.	.	.	.
Fried Rice – see Rice	...	...	.	.	.	.	.
Frosting	...	...	.	.	.	.	.
Chocolate	1 oz	120	19	0	19	0	5
Vanilla	1 oz	110	18	Tr	18	Tr	5
Frozen Dessert	...	...	.	.	.	.	.
(also see Ice Cream)	...	...	.	.	.	.	.
Ice pops 1.75 oz Regular	... 1	... 40	. 10	. 0	. 10	. 0	. Tr
w/ low calorie sweetener	1	15	3	0	3	0	0
Popsicle pops, sugarfree	1	10	3	0	3	0	0
Fudgesicle bar, fat free	1	70	14	Tr	14	3	Tr
Fudgesicle bar, no sugar added	1	90	19	1	19	3	Tr
Frozen Dinner	...	...	.	.	.	.	.
Banquet	...	...	.	.	.	.	.
Boneless Pork Ribs	1 meal	370	47	4	43	6	17
Chicken Nugget	1 meal	380	38	4	34	14	19
Crock-Pot Classics, Chicken & Dumplings	⅔ cup	200	21	6	15	10	8
Crock-Pot Classics, Hearty Beef & Vegetables	⅔ cup	140	15	4	11	12	6
Crock-Pot Classics, Meatballs in Stroganoff Sauce	⅔ cup	300	29	5	24	14	14
Fish Sticks	1 meal	360	46	3	43	13	13

	SERVING SIZE	CALORIES	TOTAL CARBS (g)	FIBER (g)	NET CARBS (g)	PROTEIN (g)	FAT (g)
Fried Beef Steak	1 meal	390	41	3	38	14	19
Meatloaf	1 meal	300	28	5	23	14	15
Original Fried Chicken	1 meal	380	35	5	30	14	20
Original Fried Chicken Meal	1 meal	430	39	4	35	21	21
Salisbury Steak	1 meal	300	25	5	20	14	16
Swedish Meatballs	1 meal	430	35	5	30	20	23
Turkey Dinner	1 meal	200	27	5	22	14	8
Healthy Choice	. . .	. . .	.	.	.	.	.
Beef Pot Roast	1 meal	260	40	7	33	14	5
Chicken Fettucini Alfredo	1 meal	290	41	7	34	16	6
Five-Spice Beef & Vegetables	1 meal	290	48	4	44	14	5
General Tso's Spicy Chicken	1 meal	320	53	4	49	15	4
Orange Zest Chicken	1 meal	290	46	6	40	17	4
Pumpkin Squash Ravioli	1 meal	300	52	6	46	9	6
Roasted Chicken Fresca	1 meal	230	29	6	23	17	5
Roasted Chicken Marsala	1 meal	250	30	4	26	18	6
Sweet Sesame Chicken	1 meal	330	50	6	44	17	6
Bacon & Smokey Cheddar Chicken	1 meal	260	32	3	29	18	6
Beef Tips Portobello	1 meal	260	34	5	29	16	6
Cajun Style Chicken & Shrimp	1 meal	260	40	3	37	15	4
Chicken Alfredo Florentine	1 meal	230	31	4	27	17	4

	SERVING SIZE	CALORIES	TOTAL CARBS (g)	FIBER (g)	NET CARBS (g)	PROTEIN (g)	FAT (g)
Chicken Margherita	1 meal	320	45	5	40	18	7
Chicken Parmigiana	1 meal	340	49	8	41	16	9
Chicken Pesto Classico	1 meal	320	39	4	35	19	9
Chicken Red Pepper Alfredo	1 meal	250	30	4	26	20	5
Classic Meat Loaf	1 meal	300	40	9	31	15	8
Country Breaded Chicken	1 meal	370	53	6	47	15	9
Country Herb Chicken	1 meal	240	34	5	29	15	5
Creamy Garlic Shrimp	1 meal	240	39	6	33	13	4
Fire Roasted Tomato Chicken	1 meal	320	48	7	41	19	5
Golden Roasted Turkey Breast	1 meal	320	49	8	41	20	5
Grilled Basil Chicken	1 meal	290	38	5	33	20	6
Grilled Chicken BBQ	1 meal	270	43	7	36	15	3
Grilled Chicken Marinara	1 meal	270	35	5	30	21	5
Grilled Chicken Monterey	1 meal	290	41	5	36	17	6
Grilled Chicken Teryaki	1 meal	280	44	8	36	15	4
Grilled Whiskey Steak	1 meal	250	34	6	28	18	4
Hearty Beef Stroganoff	1 meal	300	43	5	38	18	6
Homestyle Salisbury Steak	1 meal	290	42	8	34	16	6
Honey Balsamic Chicken	1 meal	360	59	5	54	15	7

	SERVING SIZE	CALORIES	TOTAL CARBS (g)	FIBER (g)	NET CARBS (g)	PROTEIN (g)	FAT (g)
Honey Ginger Chicken	1 meal	310	53	3	50	14	5
Lemon Pepper Fish	1 meal	310	53	5	48	13	5
Mandarin Beef Lo Mein	1 meal	360	60	8	52	16	6
Marinara Manicotti Formaggio	1 meal	350	61	8	53	13	7
Mediterranean Pasta	1 meal	360	65	12	53	13	5
Oven Roasted Chicken	1 meal	260	37	6	31	15	5
Portabella Marsala Pasta	1 meal	270	38	5	33	12	7
Portabella Spinach Parmesan	1 meal	270	40	5	35	11	7
Roasted Beef Merlot	1 meal	230	21	5	16	17	8
Roasted Sesame Chicken	1 meal	340	53	5	48	18	6
Salisbury Steak	1 meal	190	18	5	13	14	6
Slow Roasted Turkey Medallions	1 meal	220	28	5	23	14	5
Sweet & Sour Chicken	1 meal	400	61	5	56	13	10
Sweet Asian Potstickers	1 meal	380	75	6	69	8	5
Sweet Bourbon Steak Tips	1 meal	290	38	6	32	17	7
Tomato Basil Penne	1 meal	280	39	7	32	13	6
Turkey Breast & Cranberries	1 meal	320	53	7	46	16	4
Lean Cuisine	. . .	. . .	.	.	.	.	.
Alfredo Pasta w/ Chicken & Broccoli	1 meal	250	33	3	30	17	6

	SERVING SIZE	CALORIES	TOTAL CARBS (g)	FIBER (g)	NET CARBS (g)	PROTEIN (g)	FAT (g)
Angel Hair Pomodoro	1 meal	250	42	4	38	8	5
Asian Style Potstickers	1 meal	260	47	3	44	9	4
Baked Chicken	1 meal	240	34	3	31	15	5
Baked Chicken Florentine	1 meal	200	14	3	11	18	8
Balsamic Glazed Chicken	1 meal	350	43	6	37	24	9
Beef & Broccoli	1 meal	260	39	2	37	14	5
Beef Chow Fun	1 meal	320	54	3	51	15	5
Beef Portabello	1 meal	220	25	2	23	16	6
Beef Pot Roast	1 meal	210	26	3	23	14	6
Butternut Squash Ravioli	1 meal	350	54	6	48	13	9
Cheddar Potatoes w/ Broccoli	1 meal	230	35	4	31	12	5
Cheese Lasagna w/ Chicken Breast Scallopini	1 meal	280	34	4	30	18	8
Cheese Ravioli	1 meal	240	36	3	33	11	6
Chicken & Vegetables	1 meal	240	29	3	26	20	5
Chicken Carbonara	1 meal	280	33	2	31	22	7
Chicken Chow Mein	1 meal	260	41	3	38	14	4
Chicken Enchilada Suiza	1 meal	270	47	3	44	12	4
Chicken Fettuccini	1 meal	400	48	6	42	33	8
Chicken Fettuccini	1 meal	270	32	0	32	22	6
Chicken Florentine	1 meal	410	54	6	48	28	9
Chicken Florentine Lasagna	1 meal	280	36	3	33	20	6
Chicken Fried Rice Bowl	1 meal	280	39	3	36	17	6

	SERVING SIZE	CALORIES	TOTAL CARBS (g)	FIBER (g)	NET CARBS (g)	PROTEIN (g)	FAT (g)
Chicken in Peanut Sauce	1 meal	280	30	5	25	22	8
Chicken Marsala	1 meal	250	29	2	27	14	9
Chicken Mediterranean	1 meal	240	32	6	26	19	4
Chicken Parmesan	1 meal	310	39	5	34	21	8
Chicken Pecan	1 meal	260	32	4	28	19	6
Chicken Portabello	1 meal	390	48	2	46	32	8
Chicken Teriyaki Bowl	1 meal	250	44	3	41	15	2
Chicken Teriyaki Stir Fry	1 meal	250	46	3	43	12	2
Chicken Tuscan	1 meal	280	34	5	29	22	6
Chicken w/ Almonds	1 meal	260	34	3	31	17	6
Chicken w/ Basil Cream Sauce	1 meal	290	36	3	33	20	7
Classic Five Cheese Lasagna	1 meal	360	51	4	47	21	8
Classic Macaroni & Beef	1 meal	310	38	3	35	20	9
Deluxe Cheddar Potato	1 meal	260	35	4	31	14	7
Fettuccini Alfredo	1 meal	280	42	1	41	14	6
Fiesta Grilled Chicken	1 meal	260	33	4	29	19	6
Five Cheese Rigatoni	1 meal	330	50	4	46	12	9
Four Cheese Cannelloni	1 meal	240	30	3	27	17	6
Ginger Garlic Stir Fry w/ Chicken	1 meal	290	46	4	42	17	4
Glazed Chicken	1 meal	220	25	1	24	21	4

	SERVING SIZE	CALORIES	TOTAL CARBS (g)	FIBER (g)	NET CARBS (g)	PROTEIN (g)	FAT (g)
Glazed Turkey Tenderloins	1 meal	250	38	3	35	13	5
Grilled Chicken & Penne Pasta	1 meal	330	52	6	46	20	5
Grilled Chicken Caesar Bowl	1 meal	240	25	3	22	18	7
Grilled Chicken Primavera	1 meal	220	24	5	19	18	5
Grilled Chicken w/ Teriyaki Glaze	1 meal	280	45	2	43	17	3
Herb Roasted Chicken	1 meal	180	20	3	17	18	4
Honey Dijon Grilled Chicken	1 meal	220	22	2	20	17	7
Hunan Stir Fry w/ Beef	1 meal	270	37	2	35	15	7
Jumbo Rigatoni w/ Meatballs	1 meal	390	56	7	49	23	8
Lasagna w/ Meat Sauce	1 meal	320	43	4	39	20	7
Lemon Chicken	1 meal	300	41	3	38	13	9
Lemon Garlic Shrimp	1 meal	350	54	5	49	18	7
Lemon Pepper Fish	1 meal	330	50	2	48	15	8
Lemongrass Chicken	1 meal	250	30	4	26	18	6
Linguini Carbonara	1 meal	300	43	2	41	14	8
Macaroni & Cheese	1 meal	290	41	1	40	15	7
Mealoaf w/ Gravy & Whipped Potatoes	1 meal	260	25	3	22	21	8
Orange Chicken	1 meal	300	46	2	44	14	7
Orange Peel Chicken	1 meal	390	63	3	60	15	9

	SERVING SIZE	CALORIES	TOTAL CARBS (g)	FIBER (g)	NET CARBS (g)	PROTEIN (g)	FAT (g)
Oven Roasted Beef	1 meal	210	18	2	16	16	8
Oven Roasted Beef Burgundy	1 meal	300	39	3	36	17	8
Parmesan Crusted Fish	1 meal	290	40	4	36	15	8
Pasta Romano w/ Bacon	1 meal	280	43	4	39	12	7
Pesto Chicken w/ Bowtie Pasta	1 meal	340	42	4	38	23	9
Roasted Chicken w/ Lemon Pepper Fettuccini	1 meal	230	28	2	26	16	6
Roasted Garlic Chicken	1 meal	180	9	1	8	20	7
Roasted Turkey & Vegetables	1 meal	150	12	3	9	15	5
Roasted Turkey Breast	1 meal	290	38	5	33	19	7
Roasted Turkey Breast w/ Dressing	1 meal	260	48	3	45	12	3
Rosemary Chicken	1 meal	210	27	3	24	17	4
Salisbury Steak	1 meal	270	27	10	17	22	8
Salisbury Steak w/ Mac & Cheese	1 meal	280	25	3	22	24	9
Salmon Mediterranean	1 meal	230	30	3	27	18	4
Salmon w/ Basil	1 meal	220	23	4	19	19	6
Sante Fe Style Rice & Beans	1 meal	300	52	5	47	11	5
Sesame Chicken	1 meal	330	47	2	45	16	9
Sesame Stir Fry w/ Chicken	1 meal	300	41	5	36	20	6
Shrimp & Angel Hair Pasta	1 meal	220	32	2	30	14	4

	SERVING SIZE	CALORIES	TOTAL CARBS (g)	FIBER (g)	NET CARBS (g)	PROTEIN (g)	FAT (g)
Shrimp Alfredo	1 meal	260	36	3	33	18	5
Southern Beef Tips	1 meal	250	36	3	33	15	5
Spaghetti w/ Meat Sauce	1 meal	290	47	4	43	15	5
Spaghetti w/ Meatballs	1 meal	270	38	5	33	18	5
Steak Tips Dijon	1 meal	280	33	5	28	21	7
Steak Tips Portobello	1 meal	180	13	3	10	15	7
Stuffed Cabbage	1 meal	220	21	5	16	24	4
Sun Dried Tomato Pesto Chicken	1 meal	290	34	4	30	18	9
Swedish Meatballs	1 meal	300	34	3	31	22	8
Sweet & Sour Chicken	1 meal	310	53	2	51	17	3
Szechuan Style Stir Fry w/ Shrimp	1 meal	230	39	5	34	13	3
Teriyaki Steak Bowl	1 meal	280	37	3	34	19	6
Thai-Style Chicken	1 meal	220	28	2	26	18	4
Three Cheese Chicken	1 meal	210	10	3	7	21	10
Three Cheese Stuffed Rigatoni Bowl	1 meal	240	35	4	31	12	6
Tortilla Crusted Fish	1 meal	330	45	3	42	16	9
Vegetable Eggroll	1 meal	310	60	3	57	7	5
Marie Callender's	...	...	.	.	.	.	.
Beef Tips Dinner	1 meal	360	35	6	29	26	12
Cheesy Chicken Breast, Rice w/ Broccoli	1 meal	480	47	5	42	31	18
Fettuccine Chicken & Broccoli	1 meal	630	43	6	37	30	37

	SERVING SIZE	CALORIES	TOTAL CARBS (g)	FIBER (g)	NET CARBS (g)	PROTEIN (g)	FAT (g)
Grilled Chicken Bake	1 meal	610	43	5	38	30	35
Herb Roasted Chicken	1 meal	460	26	5	21	30	25
Meat Loaf w/ Gravy	1 meal	480	39	3	36	31	22
Old Fashioned Beef Pot Roast	1 meal	330	32	9	23	27	10
Salisbury Steak Dinner	1 meal	400	38	7	31	27	16
Slow Roasted Beef	1 meal	370	37	7	30	25	13
Turkey w/ Stuffing	1 meal	400	45	4	41	32	9
Smart Ones (Weight Watchers)	...	...	.	.	.	.	.
Angel Hair Marinara	1 meal	230	40	4	36	9	4
Broccoli & Cheddar Roasted Potatoes	1 meal	240	35	4	31	10	7
Chicken Carbonara	1 meal	250	32	2	30	20	5
Chicken Enchiladas Monterey	1 meal	310	41	5	36	12	10
Chicken Enchiladas Suiza	1 meal	290	49	3	46	11	5
Chicken Fettuccini	1 meal	340	47	4	43	23	6
Chicken Marsala w/ Broccoli	1 meal	180	10	2	8	20	7
Chicken Mirabella	1 meal	200	33	3	30	12	2
Chicken Oriental	1 meal	230	39	2	37	12	3
Chicken Parmesan	1 meal	290	35	4	31	26	5
Chicken Santa Fe	1 meal	140	11	4	7	20	3
Cranberry Turkey Medallions	1 meal	250	43	4	39	16	2
Creamy Parmesan Chicken	1 meal	250	24	3	21	21	8

FOODS | 101

	SERVING SIZE	CALORIES	TOTAL CARBS (g)	FIBER (g)	NET CARBS (g)	PROTEIN (g)	FAT (g)
Creamy Rigatoni w/ Chicken & Broccoli	1 meal	290	33	2	31	20	8
Dragon Shrimp Lo Mein	1 meal	240	36	3	33	14	4
Fettucini Alfredo	1 meal	240	41	4	37	12	4
Home Style Beef Pot Roast	1 meal	180	20	3	17	17	5
Honey Mango Barbeque Chicken	1 meal	240	34	0	34	9	4
Lasagna Bake w/ Meat Sauce	1 meal	270	43	3	40	14	4
Lasagna Florentine	1 meal	290	35	4	29	15	9
Lemon Herb Chicken Piccata	1 meal	230	41	2	39	12	2
Macaroni & Cheese	1 meal	270	52	2	50	11	2
Meatloaf	1 meal	250	23	3	20	22	8
Orange Sesame Chicken	1 meal	320	48	2	46	14	8
Pasta Primavera	1 meal	280	44	6	38	12	6
Picante Chicken & Pasta	1 meal	260	32	4	28	23	4
Pineapple Beef Teriyaki	1 meal	260	38	0	38	18	5
Ravioli Florentine	1 meal	250	40	4	36	11	5
Roast Beef w/ Gravy	1 meal	210	19	2	17	14	9
Roast Turkey Medallions w/ Mushroom Gravy	1 meal	220	38	3	35	13	2
Roasted Chicken w/ Sour Cream & Chive Mashed Potatoes	1 meal	180	20	2	18	17	4

	SERVING SIZE	CALORIES	TOTAL CARBS (g)	FIBER (g)	NET CARBS (g)	PROTEIN (g)	FAT (g)
Salisbury Steak	1 meal	200	12	3	9	20	8
Santa Fe Style Rice & Beans	1 meal	310	51	4	47	10	7
Shrimp Marinara	1 meal	180	31	4	27	9	2
Sirloin Beef & Asian Style Vegetables	1 meal	220	27	3	24	17	5
Slow Roasted Turkey Breast	1 meal	210	18	2	16	18	7
Spaghetti w/ Meat Sauce	1 meal	310	48	5	43	16	6
Spicy Szechuan Style Vegetable & Chicken	1 meal	240	36	4	32	11	5
Stuffed Turkey Breast	1 meal	290	42	4	38	17	6
Swedish Meatballs	1 meal	270	35	3	32	20	5
Sweet & Sour Chicken	1 meal	210	31	2	29	16	2
Teriyaki Chicken & Vegetables	1 meal	230	39	3	36	14	3
Thai Style Chicken & Rice Noodles	1 meal	260	43	2	41	14	4
Three Cheese Macaroni	1 meal	300	48	3	45	14	6
Three Cheese Ziti Marinara	1 meal	320	47	4	43	14	8
Traditional Lasagna w/ Meat Sauce	1 meal	300	43	5	38	17	6
Tuna Noodle Gratin	1 meal	240	37	3	34	15	5
Turkey Medallions w/ Mushroom Gravy	1 meal	200	11	3	8	18	10

	SERVING SIZE	CALORIES	TOTAL CARBS (g)	FIBER (g)	NET CARBS (g)	PROTEIN (g)	FAT (g)
Stouffers	. . .	. . .	.	.	.	.	.
Macaroni & Beef	1 meal	410	45	4	41	22	16
Baked Chicken Breast	1 meal	250	20	1	19	20	10
Beef Pot Roast	1 meal	320	41	8	33	20	8
Beef Stroganoff	1 meal	380	34	2	32	22	17
Bourbon Steak Tips	1 meal	570	65	4	61	23	24
Cheese Manicotti	1 meal	360	41	2	39	18	14
Cheese Ravioli	1 meal	380	47	5	42	19	13
Cheesy Spaghetti Bake	1 meal	460	39	4	35	21	24
Chicken a la King	1 meal	360	44	0	44	18	12
Chicken Carbonara	1 meal	670	56	6	50	40	32
Chicken Fettuccini	1 meal	570	55	5	50	26	27
Chicken Fettuccini Alfredo	1 meal	840	94	5	89	31	38
Chicken Parmigiana	1 meal	410	47	4	43	23	14
Escalloped Chicken & Noodles	1 meal	450	43	5	38	19	22
Fettuccini Alfredo	1 meal	610	57	5	52	18	34
Fish Filet	1 meal	400	36	4	32	27	16
Five Cheese Lasagna	1 meal	370	39	4	35	21	14
Fried Chicken Breast	1 meal	360	30	2	28	20	18
Garlic Chicken Pasta	1 meal	330	37	5	32	25	9
Green Pepper Steak	1 meal	240	32	3	29	18	4
Grilled Chicken Teriyaki	1 meal	300	45	3	42	21	4

	SERVING SIZE	CALORIES	TOTAL CARBS (g)	FIBER (g)	NET CARBS (g)	PROTEIN (g)	FAT (g)
Grilled Herb Chicken	1 meal	250	29	3	26	19	6
Grilled Lemon Pepper Chicken	1 meal	240	24	4	20	19	8
Lasagna Bake w/ Meat Sauce	1 meal	350	49	5	44	17	10
Lasagna w/ Meat & Sauce	1 meal	350	38	3	35	24	11
Lasagna w/ Tomato Sauce & Italian Sausage	1 meal	410	41	4	37	18	19
Macaroni & Cheese w/ Broccoli	1 meal	480	52	5	47	22	20
Meatloaf	1 meal	600	45	5	40	35	31
Monterey Chicken	1 meal	530	54	5	49	31	21
Pork Cutlet	1 meal	370	31	3	28	13	21
Rigatoni w/ Roasted White Chicken Meat	1 meal	390	44	3	41	19	15
Roast Turkey	1 meal	290	30	2	28	16	12
Roast Turkey Breast	1 meal	460	51	5	46	22	19
Roasted Chicken	1 meal	460	34	5	29	26	24
Salisbury Steak	1 meal	710	48	3	45	41	39
Sesame Chicken	1 meal	590	87	6	81	25	16
Shrimp Scampi	1 meal	400	56	5	51	16	12
Spaghetti w/ Meat Sauce	1 meal	350	44	5	39	17	12
Spaghetti w/ Meatballs	1 meal	360	45	6	39	19	12
Swedish Meatballs	1 meal	560	47	3	44	32	27
Tuna Noodle Casserole	1 meal	450	45	3	42	22	20
Turkey Tetrazzini	1 meal	450	38	2	36	23	23

	SERVING SIZE	CALORIES	TOTAL CARBS (g)	FIBER (g)	NET CARBS (g)	PROTEIN (g)	FAT (g)
Veal Parmigiana	1 meal	430	46	5	41	20	18
Vegetable Lasagna	1 meal	390	40	4	36	17	18
Stuffed Pepper	1 meal	210	23	3	20	10	9
Fruit (see specific listings)	...	...	.	.	.	.	.
Mixed, canned, in heavy syrup	1 cup	180	48	3	45	Tr	Tr
Mixed, frozen, sweetened	1 cup	250	61	5	56	4	Tr
Fruit Cocktail	...	...	.	.	.	.	.
Canned in heavy syrup	1 cup	180	47	3	42	Tr	Tr
Canned in light syrup	1 cup	140	36	2	34	Tr	Tr
Canned in juice	1 cup	110	28	2	26	1	Tr
Fruit Salad	...	...	.	.	.	.	.
Canned in heavy syrup	1 cup	190	49	3	46	Tr	Tr
Canned in light syrup	1 cup	150	38	3	35	Tr	Tr
Canned in juice	1 cup	130	33	3	30	1	Tr
Tropical, canned in heavy syrup	1 cup	220	58	3	55	1	Tr
Fudge-see Candy	...	...	.	.	.	.	.
Funyuns (snacks)	13	140	18	1	17	2	7
Garlic, raw	1 clove	0	Tr	Tr	Tr	Tr	Tr
Garlic Powder or Salt	1 tsp	10	2	Tr	2	Tr	Tr
Gelatin (*Jello*)	...	...	.	.	.	.	.
unsweetened, 1 envelope	1 Tbsp	25	0	0	0	6	Tr
sweetened w/sugar, as prep	½ cup	80	19	0	19	2	0
reduced calorie, sweetened w/ aspartame, as prep	½ cup	25	5	0	5	Tr	0

	SERVING SIZE	CALORIES	TOTAL CARBS (g)	FIBER (g)	NET CARBS (g)	PROTEIN (g)	FAT (g)
Ginger, dried, ground	1 tsp	5	1	Tr	1	Tr	Tr
Ginger root, fresh, grated	1 tsp	0	Tr	0	Tr	Tr	Tr
Slices, 1" dia	5	10	2	Tr	2	Tr	Tr
Gordita – see frozen dinner/individual restaurant listings	...	...	.	.	.	.	.
Granola Bar	...	...	.	.	.	.	.
Hard	...	...	.	.	.	.	.
Almond	1 oz	140	18	1	17	2	7
Peanut	1 oz	140	18	1	17	3	6
Peanut butter	1 oz	140	18	Tr	18	3	7
Plain	1 oz	130	18	2	16	3	6
Chocolate chip	1 oz	120	20	1	19	2	5
Soft	...	...	.	.	.	.	.
Chocolate chip	1 oz	120	20	1	19	2	5
Chocolate covered chocolate chip	1 oz	130	18	1	17	2	7
Chocolate covered peanut butter	1 oz	140	15	Tr	15	3	9
Nut & raisin	1 oz	130	18	2	16	2	6
Peanut butter	1 oz	120	18	1	17	3	4
Peanut butter & chocolate chip	1 oz	120	17	1	16	3	6
Plain	1 oz	130	19	1	18	2	5
Chocolate covered coconut	1 oz	150	16	2	14	2	9
Nonfat, fruit-filled	1 oz	100	22	2	20	2	Tr
Oats, fruit, & nuts	1 oz	110	22	2	20	2	2
Grapefruit, pink, red, or white	...	...	.	.	.	.	.
fresh, 4" dia	1 half	40	10	1	9	Tr	Tr
fresh, sections	1 cup	70	19	3	16	2	Tr

	SERVING SIZE	CALORIES	TOTAL CARBS (g)	FIBER (g)	NET CARBS (g)	PROTEIN (g)	FAT (g)
canned, in juice	1 cup	90	23	1	22	2	Tr
canned, in light syrup	1 cup	150	39	1	38	1	Tr
Grapes, seeded	…	…	.	.	.	.	.
Fresh, medium size, all types	10 grapes	35	9	Tr	9	Tr	Tr
Fresh, medium size, all types	1 cup	100	27	1	26	1	Tr
Gravy	…	…	.	.	.	.	.
Canned	…	…	.	.	.	.	.
Au jus	¼ cup	10	2	0	2	Tr	Tr
Beef	¼ cup	30	3	Tr	3	2	1
Chicken	¼ cup	45	3	Tr	3	1	3
Mushroom	¼ cup	30	3	Tr	3	Tr	2
Turkey	¼ cup	30	3	Tr	3	2	1
Low sodium, meat or poultry	¼ cup	30	4	Tr	4	2	1
Grits, corn, as prep	1 cup	140	31	Tr	31	3	Tr
Ground Beef – see Beef	…	…	.	.	.	.	.
Guava	…	…	.	.	.	.	.
Fresh, whole	1	35	8	3	5	1	Tr
Fresh, chopped	1 cup	110	24	9	15	4	2
Strawberry guava, whole	1	0	1	Tr	1	Tr	Tr
Gum – see Chewing Gum	…	…	.	.	.	.	.
HAM (also see Pork)	…	…	.	.	.	.	.
Canned, roasted	3 oz	190	Tr	0	Tr	18	13
extra lean, roasted	3 oz	120	Tr	0	Tr	18	4
Leg, roasted, lean & fat	3 oz	230	0	0	0	23	15
lean only	3 oz	180	0	0	0	25	8

	SERVING SIZE	CALORIES	TOTAL CARBS (g)	FIBER (g)	NET CARBS (g)	PROTEIN (g)	FAT (g)
Cured, roasted, lean & fat	3 oz	210	0	0	0	18	14
lean only	3 oz	130	0	0	0	21	5
Lunch meat, ⅛" slices	…	…	.	.	.	.	.
regular	2 oz	90	2	Tr	2	9	5
extra lean	2 oz	60	Tr	0	Tr	11	2
Steak, cured, extra lean, 1 slice	2 oz	70	0	0	0	11	2
Boarshead	…	…	.	.	.	.	.
Black Forest Brand Smoked	2 oz	60	2	0	2	10	1
Branded Deluxe Ham	2 oz	60	2	0	2	9	1
Canadian Style Bacon, Extra Lean	2 oz	70	1	0	1	12	2
Cappy Brand Ham	2 oz	60	3	0	3	10	2
Seasoned Fresh Ham	2 oz	80	0	0	0	14	3
Smoked Virginia Ham	2 oz	60	2	0	2	9	1
Oscar Mayer	…	…	.	.	.	.	.
Chopped, 1 slice	1 oz	50	1	0	1	5	3
Baked, 96% fat free, 3 slices	2.25 oz	70	1	0	1	10	2
Baked	2.25 oz	70	Tr	0	Tr	11	2
Honey	2.25 oz	70	2	0	2	11	2
Smoked	2.25 oz	60	Tr	0	Tr	11	2
Hamburger & Cheeseburger – see Beef – Ground & Fast Food Restaurants	…	…	.	.	.	.	.

	SERVING SIZE	CALORIES	TOTAL CARBS (g)	FIBER (g)	NET CARBS (g)	PROTEIN (g)	FAT (g)
Hash Browns - see Potatoes	...	...	.	.	.	.	.
Hearts of Palm, canned	1 cup	40	7	4	3	4	Tr
Honey	1 Tbsp	60	17	0	17	Tr	0
	½ oz	40	12	0	12	Tr	0
Honeydew Melon	...	...	.	.	.	.	.
Fresh, avg size 6 ½" melon,	...	...	.	.	.	.	.
cubed or balls	1 cup	60	16	1	15	Tr	Tr
wedge, ⅛ of melon	1	60	15	1	14	Tr	Tr
Horseradish, as prep	1 tsp	0	Tr	Tr	Tr	Tr	Tr
Hot Dog (Frankfurter)	...	...	.	.	.	.	.
Beef	1	150	2	0	2	5	13
Beef, lowfat	1	130	Tr	0	Tr	7	11
Beef & pork	1	140	Tr	0	Tr	5	13
Beef & pork, lowfat	1	90	3	0	3	6	6
Chicken	1	100	1	Tr	1	7	7
Pork	1	200	Tr	Tr	Tr	10	18
Turkey	1	100	2	0	2	6	8
Boarshead	...	...	.	.	.	.	.
Lite Beef Frankfurters	1 frank	90	0	0	0	7	6
Pork and Beef Frankfurters	1 frank	150	0	0	0	7	14
Hummus, commercial	1 Tbsp	25	2	Tr	2	1	1
Hush Puppies	1	70	10	Tr	10	2	3
Ice Cream	...	...	.	.	.	.	.
Chocolate	...	...	.	.	.	.	.
regular	½ cup	140	19	Tr	19	3	7
light	½ cup	140	18	Tr	18	3	5
light, no sugar added	½ cup	110	18	Tr	18	3	4

	SERVING SIZE	CALORIES	TOTAL CARBS (g)	FIBER (g)	NET CARBS (g)	PROTEIN (g)	FAT (g)
rich	½ cup	190	15	Tr	15	4	13
Vanilla	...	...	.	.	.	.	.
regular	½ cup	140	16	Tr	16	2	7
light	½ cup	130	20	Tr	20	4	4
light, no sugar added	½ cup	110	15	Tr	15	3	5
rich	½ cup	270	24	0	24	4	17
soft-serve	½ cup	190	19	Tr	19	4	11
soft-serve, light	½ cup	110	19	0	19	4	2
Low carb	...	...	.	.	.	.	.
chocolate	½ cup	130	11	3	8	3	8
vanilla	½ cup	130	11	3	8	2	8
Sherbet, Orange	½ cup	110	23	1	22	Tr	2
Strawberry	½ cup	130	18	Tr	18	2	6
Ice Cream Cone, cake or wafer	1	15	3	Tr	3	Tr	Tr
Sugar cone	1	40	8	Tr	8	Tr	Tr
Waffle cone, large	1	120	23	Tr	23	2	2
Ice Cream Sandwich, vanilla	1	220	31	1	30	4	9
Ice Pop – See Frozen Dessert	...	...	.	.	.	.	.
Italian Ices	½ cup	60	16	0	16	Tr	Tr
Jalapeno – see Peppers	...	...	.	.	.	.	.
Jam, all flavors	...	...	.	.	.	.	.
Regular	1 Tbsp	60	14	Tr	14	Tr	Tr
Restaurant size packet	½ oz	40	10	Tr	10	Tr	Tr
Sweetened w/ sodium saccarin	1 Tbsp	20	8	Tr	8	Tr	Tr
Jello – see Gelatin	...	...	.	.	.	.	.

	SERVING SIZE	CALORIES	TOTAL CARBS (g)	FIBER (g)	NET CARBS (g)	PROTEIN (g)	FAT (g)
Jelly	...	...	.	.	.	.	.
All flavors, regular	1 Tbsp	60	15	Tr	15	Tr	0
Reduced sugar	1 Tbsp	35	9	Tr	9	Tr	Tr
Restaurant size packet	½ oz	35	10	Tr	10	Tr	0
Kale	...	...	.	.	.	.	.
Fresh, chopped	1 cup	35	7	1	6	2	Tr
Fresh, chopped, cooked	1 cup	35	7	3	4	3	Tr
Frozen, chopped, cooked	1 cup	40	7	3	4	4	Tr
Ketchup, regular	1 Tbsp	15	4	0	4	Tr	Tr
Restaurant size packet	1 pkt	5	2	0	2	Tr	Tr
Low sodium	1 Tbsp	15	4	0	4	Tr	Tr
Kiwi fruit, fresh, medium size	1	45	11	2	9	Tr	Tr
Knockwurst	1 link	220	2	0	2	8	20
Kohlrabi, cooked, slices	1 cup	50	11	2	9	3	Tr
Lamb	...	...	.	.	.	.	.
Cubed, braised	3 oz	190	0	0	0	29	8
Cubed, broiled	3 oz	160	0	0	0	24	6
Ground, broiled	3 oz	240	0	0	0	21	17
Leg of lamb, roasted	...	...	.	.	.	.	.
lean & fat	3 oz	240	0	0	0	26	14
lean only	3 oz	160	0	0	0	24	7
Loin chop, broiled	...	...	.	.	.	.	.
lean & fat	3 oz	250	0	0	0	22	18
lean only	3 oz	180	0	0	0	26	8
Rib roast, lean & fat	3 oz	290	0	0	0	19	23
lean only	3 oz	200	0	0	0	22	11

	SERVING SIZE	CALORIES	TOTAL CARBS (g)	FIBER (g)	NET CARBS (g)	PROTEIN (g)	FAT (g)
Shoulder, brasied	...	...	.	.	.	.	.
lean & fat	3 oz	290	0	0	0	25	20
lean only	3 oz	240	0	0	0	28	14
Lard	1 cup	1850	0	0	0	0	205
	1 Tbsp	120	0	0	0	0	13
Lasagna, 1 piece	...	...	.	.	.	.	.
w/ meat sauce	1	380	38	4	34	25	14
vegetable	1	320	32	4	28	16	14
Leek, chopped, cooked	¼ cup	10	2	Tr	2	Tr	Tr
Whole, cooked	1	40	10	1	9	1	Tr
Lemon, fresh, 2 ¼" dia	1	20	12	5	7	1	Tr
Lentils, cooked	½ cup	120	20	8	12	9	Tr
Lettuce, fresh, raw	...	...	.	.	.	.	.
Bibb, Boston, Butterhead	...	...	.	.	.	.	.
whole head, 5" dia	1	20	4	2	2	2	Tr
single leaf	1	0	Tr	Tr	Tr	Tr	Tr
Green leaf	...	...	.	.	.	.	.
whole head	1	50	10	5	5	5	Tr
inner leaf	1	0	Tr	Tr	Tr	Tr	Tr
pieces, shredded	1 cup	5	1	Tr	1	Tr	Tr
Iceberg, Crisphead	...	.	.	.	.	.	Tr
whole head, 6" dia	1	80	16	7	9	5	Tr
single leaf	1	0	Tr	Tr	Tr	Tr	Tr
pieces, shredded	1 cup	10	2	Tr	2	Tr	Tr
wedge slice, ⅙ of 6" head	1	15	3	1	2	Tr	Tr
Red leaf	...	...	.	.	.	.	.
whole head	1	50	7	3	4	4	Tr

	SERVING SIZE	CALORIES	TOTAL CARBS (g)	FIBER (g)	NET CARBS (g)	PROTEIN (g)	FAT (g)
inner leaf	1	0	Tr	0	Tr	Tr	Tr
pieces, shredded	1 cup	0	Tr	Tr	Tr	Tr	Tr
Romaine or cos	...	...	.	.	.	.	.
whole head	1	110	21	13	8	8	2
inner leaf	1	0	Tr	Tr	Tr	Tr	Tr
pieces, shredded	1 cup	10	2	1	1	Tr	Tr
Lime, fresh, 2" dia	1	20	7	2	5	Tr	Tr
Liver	...	...	.	.	.	.	.
Beef liver, fried	3 oz	150	4	0	4	23	4
Chicken livers, simmered	3 oz	140	Tr	0	Tr	21	6
Veal liver, braised	3 oz	160	3	0	3	24	5
Liverwurst, pork	2 oz	190	1	0	1	8	16
Lobster – see Fish / Seafood	...	...	.	.	.	.	.
Lunch Meat (thin ⅛" slices)	...	...	.	.	.	.	.
Beef or Pork, regular	2 slices	200	1	0	1	7	18
Chicken, roasted	2 slices	35	Tr	0	Tr	7	Tr
Chicken, smoked	2 slices	35	Tr	0	Tr	7	Tr
Turkey, regular	2 slices	45	2	0	2	7	Tr
Ham, regular	2 slices	90	2	Tr	2	9	5
Ham, extra lean	2 slices	60	Tr	0	Tr	10	1
(also see specific listings)	...	.	.	.	.	.	.
Macaroni, elbows	...	...	.	.	.	.	.
Plain, cooked	1 cup	220	43	3	40	8	1
Whole wheat, cooked	1 cup	170	37	4	33	8	Tr
Macaroni & Cheese	1 cup	300	40	3	37	10	10
Mackerel – see Fish	...	...	.	.	.	.	.

	SERVING SIZE	CALORIES	TOTAL CARBS (g)	FIBER (g)	NET CARBS (g)	PROTEIN (g)	FAT (g)
Malt O Meal-see Cereal	...	...	.	.	.	.	.
Mandarin Oranges	...	...	.	.	.	.	.
Fresh, whole, 2 ½″	1	45	12	2	10	Tr	Tr
Fresh, sections	1 cup	100	26	4	22	2	Tr
Canned, in juice	1 cup	70	18	2	16	1	Tr
Canned in light syrup	1 cup	150	41	2	39	1	Tr
Mango	...	...	.	.	.	.	.
Fresh, whole	1	140	35	4	31	1	Tr
Fresh, peeled, sliced	1 cup	110	28	3	25	Tr	Tr
Margarine	...	...	.	.	.	.	.
Regular, 4 sticks/Lb	1 stick	810	Tr	0	Tr	Tr	91
Regular, hard or soft	1 cup	1630	2	0	2	Tr	183
Regular, hard or soft	1 Tbsp	100	Tr	0	Tr	Tr	11
Regular, hard or soft	1 pat	35	Tr	0	Tr	Tr	4
Fat free	1 cup	100	10	0	10	Tr	7
Fat free	1 Tbsp	5	Tr	0	Tr	Tr	Tr
Vegetable oil spread, 60% fat	1 cup	1220	2	0	2	Tr	137
Vegetable oil spread, 60% fat	1 Tbsp	80	Tr	0	Tr	Tr	8
Vegetable oil spread, 20% fat	1 cup	420	Tr	0	Tr	0	47
Vegetable oil spread, 20% fat	1 Tbsp	25	Tr	0	Tr	0	3
Marjoram, dried spice	1 tsp	0	Tr	Tr	Tr	Tr	Tr
Marmalade	1 Tbsp	50	13	Tr	13	Tr	0
	½ oz	35	9	Tr	9	Tr	0
Marshmallow	...	...	.	.	.	.	.
Miniature size	1 cup	160	41	Tr	41	Tr	Tr
Regular size	1	25	6	0	6	Tr	Tr

	SERVING SIZE	CALORIES	TOTAL CARBS (g)	FIBER (g)	NET CARBS (g)	PROTEIN (g)	FAT (g)
Marshmallow Topping	1 oz	90	22	0	22	Tr	Tr
Mayonnaise	...	...	.	.	.	.	.
Regular	1 Tbsp	100	Tr	0	Tr	Tr	11
Regular	1 cup	1580	7	0	7	2	175
Dressing, no cholesterol	1 Tbsp	100	Tr	0	Tr	0	12
Light / reduced calorie	1 Tbsp	50	1	0	1	Tr	5
Fat free	1 Tbsp	15	3	Tr	3	Tr	Tr
Meat – see specific listings	...	...	.	.	.	.	.
Meatless Burger – see Vegetable or Soy Burger	...	...	.	.	.	.	.
Meatloaf – see Frozen Dinner	...	...	.	.	.	.	.
Meatloaf, vegetarian	1 slice	110	5	3	2	12	5
Minestrone – see Soup	...	...	.	.	.	.	.
Molasses	1 Tbsp	60	15	0	15	0	Tr
	1 cup	980	252	0	252	0	Tr
Mortadella	1 slice	50	Tr	0	Tr	3	4
Muffin, sm size, 2¾" dia	...	...	.	.	.	.	.
Plain	1	170	24	2	22	4	7
Oat bran	1	180	32	3	29	5	5
Blueberry	1	260	33	1	32	4	13
Blueberry, lowfat	1	180	36	3	33	3	3
Corn	1	200	34	2	32	4	6
(also see English Muffin)	...	...	.	.	.	.	.

	SERVING SIZE	CALORIES	TOTAL CARBS (g)	FIBER (g)	NET CARBS (g)	PROTEIN (g)	FAT (g)
Mulberries	1 cup	60	14	2	12	2	Tr
Mushrooms	...	...	.	.	.	.	.
Regular, white button	...	...	.	.	.	.	.
Canned, drained solids	1 cup	40	8	4	4	3	Tr
Diced	1 cup	20	4	1	3	2	Tr
Dried, whole	4	45	11	2	9	1	Tr
Fresh, cooked, pieces	1 cup	80	21	3	18	2	Tr
Fresh, raw, slices	1 cup	15	2	Tr	2	2	Tr
Fresh, sliced, cooked	1 cup	45	8	3	5	3	Tr
Grilled, sliced	1 cup	40	6	3	3	5	Tr
Whole	1	20	4	1	3	2	Tr
Crimini, sliced	1 cup	20	3	Tr	3	2	Tr
Enoki, whole	1 cup	30	5	2	3	2	Tr
Maitake, diced	1 cup	25	5	2	3	1	Tr
Oyster, sliced	1 cup	35	6	2	4	3	Tr
Portabello	...	...	.	.	.	.	.
Shiitake	...	...	.	.	.	.	.
Straw, canned, drained	1 cup	60	8	5	3	7	1
Mussels – see Fish/Seafood	...	...	.	.	.	.	.
Mustard, yellow	1 tsp	0	Tr	Tr	Tr	Tr	Tr
Mustard seed, yellow	1 tsp	15	1	Tr	1	Tr	Tr
Mustard Greens	...	...	.	.	.	.	.
Chopped, cooked	1 cup	20	3	3	0	3	Tr
Frozen, chopped, cooked	1 cup	30	5	4	1	3	Tr
Nectarine, fresh, med, 2 ½" dia	1	60	15	2	13	2	Tr
Fresh, sliced	1 cup	60	15	2	13	2	Tr

	SERVING SIZE	CALORIES	TOTAL CARBS (g)	FIBER (g)	NET CARBS (g)	PROTEIN (g)	FAT (g)
Noodles	...	...	.	.	.	.	.
Egg noodles	...	...	.	.	.	.	.
Dry, uncooked	1 cup	150	27	1	26	5	2
Plain, cooked	1 cup	220	40	2	38	7	3
Chow Mein noodles	1 cup	240	26	2	24	4	14
Rice noodles, cooked	1 cup	190	44	2	42	2	Tr
Spinach noodles, dry	1 cup	150	27	3	24	6	2
Spinach noodles, cooked	1 cup	210	39	4	35	8	3
Nuts	...	...	.	.	.	.	.
Almonds	...	...	.	.	.	.	.
whole, about 23	1 oz	160	6	4	2	6	14
sliced almonds	¼ cup	130	5	3	2	5	11
blanched, whole	1 oz	170	6	3	3	6	14
dry roasted, whole	1 oz	170	6	3	3	6	15
honey roasted, whole	1 oz	170	8	4	4	5	14
Brazil nuts, whole, about 6	1 oz	190	4	2	2	4	19
Cashews, whole, dry roasted, about 18	1 oz	160	9	Tr	9	4	13
Chestnuts, roasted, shelled, about 3	1 oz	70	15	1	14	Tr	Tr
Coconut-see Coconut	...	...	.	.	.	.	.
Hazelnuts, about 21	1 oz	180	5	3	2	4	17
Macadamia nuts, about 11	1 oz	200	4	2	2	2	22
Mixed Nuts w/ peanuts, dry roasted	1 oz	170	7	3	4	5	15
Mixed Nuts w/ peanuts, oil roasted	1 oz	180	6	3	3	5	16

	SERVING SIZE	CALORIES	TOTAL CARBS (g)	FIBER (g)	NET CARBS (g)	PROTEIN (g)	FAT (g)
Mixed Nuts w/o peanuts, oil roasted	1 oz	170	6	2	4	4	16
Peanuts	. . .	. . .	.	.	.	.	.
boiled	1 oz	90	6	3	3	4	6
dry roasted	1 cup	850	31	12	19	35	73
dry roasted	1 oz	170	6	2	4	7	14
oil roasted	1 oz	170	5	2	3	8	14
Pecan halves, about 19	1 oz	200	4	3	1	3	20
Pine nuts	1 oz	190	4	1	3	4	19
Pistachio nuts, shelled, about 49	1 oz	160	8	3	5	6	13
Walnuts, English	. . .	. . .	.	.	.	.	.
chopped	¼ cup	190	4	2	2	5	19
halves, about 14	1 oz	190	4	2	2	4	19
Nut Butter	. . .	. . .	.	.	.	.	.
Almond	1 Tbsp	100	3	Tr	3	2	10
Cashew	1 Tbsp	90	4	Tr	4	3	8
Peanut-see Peanut Butter	. . .	. . .	.	.	.	.	.
Oat Bran	. . .	. . .	.	.	.	.	.
Uncooked	1 cup	230	62	15	47	16	7
Cooked	1 cup	90	25	6	19	7	2
Oatmeal, plain, as prep w/ water	¾ cup	120	21	3	18	5	3
Oats	1 cup	610	103	17	86	26	11
OIL (for cooking & salads)	. . .	. . .	.	.	.	.	.
PAM cooking spray, ⅓ second spray	1	0	0	0	0	0	0
Canola oil	1 cup	1930	0	0	0	0	218
Canola oil	Tbsp	120	0	0	0	0	14

	SERVING SIZE	CALORIES	TOTAL CARBS (g)	FIBER (g)	NET CARBS (g)	PROTEIN (g)	FAT (g)
Corn oil	1 cup	1930	0	0	0	0	218
Corn oil	Tbsp	120	0	0	0	0	14
Cottonseed/soybean oil blend	1 cup	1930	0	0	0	0	218
Cottonseed/soybean oil blend	1 Tbsp	120	0	0	0	0	14
Olive oil	1 cup	1910	0	0	0	0	216
Olive oil	1 Tbsp	120	0	0	0	0	14
Peanut oil	1 cup	1910	0	0	0	0	216
Peanut oil	1 Tbsp	120	0	0	0	0	14
Safflower oil	1 cup	1930	0	0	0	0	218
Safflower oil	1 Tbsp	120	0	0	0	0	14
Sesame oil	1 cup	1930	0	0	0	0	218
Sesame oil	1 Tbsp	120	0	0	0	0	14
Soybean oil	1 cup	1930	0	0	0	0	218
Soybean oil	1 Tbsp	120	0	0	0	0	14
Sunflower oil	1 cup	1930	0	0	0	0	218
Sunflower oil	1 Tbsp	120	0	0	0	0	14
Vegetable oil (grapeseed)	1 cup	1930	0	0	0	0	218
Vegetable oil (grapeseed)	1 Tbsp	120	0	0	0	0	14
Okra	. . .	. . .	.	.	.	.	.
Fresh, sliced, cooked	½ cup	20	4	2	2	2	Tr
Frozen, slices, cooked	½ cup	25	5	3	2	2	Tr
Whole, 3" pods, cooked	8 pods	20	4	2	2	2	Tr
Olive	. . .	. . .	.	.	.	.	.
Pickled, green, med size	5	20	Tr	Tr	Tr	Tr	2
Black, canned, lg size	5	25	1	Tr	1	Tr	2

	SERVING SIZE	CALORIES	TOTAL CARBS (g)	FIBER (g)	NET CARBS (g)	PROTEIN (g)	FAT (g)
Olive Loaf, 2 slices	2 oz	130	5	0	5	7	9
Onion	...	...	.	.	.	.	.
Round yellow or white onion	...	...	.	.	.	.	.
Fresh, raw, whole, 2 ½″ dia	1	45	10	2	8	1	Tr
Fresh, chopped	1 cup	60	15	3	12	2	Tr
Fresh, sliced, ⅛″ thick	1 slice	5	1	Tr	1	Tr	Tr
Frozen, cooked, boiled, whole	1 cup	60	14	3	11	2	Tr
Cooked, boiled, whole, 2 ½″ dia	1	40	10	1	9	1	Tr
Cooked, boiled, sliced or chopped	1 cup	90	21	3	18	3	Tr
Cooked, sauteed, chopped	1 cup	120	7	2	5	Tr	9
Spring onion w/ green tops & bulbs	...	...	.	.	.	.	.
Fresh, chopped	1 whole	10	2	Tr	2	Tr	Tr
Fresh, chopped	1 cup	30	7	3	4	2	Tr
Fresh, tops only, chopped	1 Tbsp	0	Tr	Tr	Tr	Tr	Tr
Sweet onion, raw	1 whole	110	25	3	22	3	Tr
Onion Flakes, dried	1 Tbsp	15	4	Tr	4	Tr	Tr
Onion Powder or Salt	1 tsp	10	2	Tr	2	Tr	Tr
Onion Rings	...	...	.	.	.	.	.
Breaded, fried, med sized	5 rings	120	12	Tr	12	2	8
Orange	...	...	.	.	.	.	.
Fresh, large size, 3″ dia	1	90	22	4	18	2	Tr
Fresh, sections	1 cup	90	21	4	17	2	Tr

	SERVING SIZE	CALORIES	TOTAL CARBS (g)	FIBER (g)	NET CARBS (g)	PROTEIN (g)	FAT (g)
Oregano, dried, leaves	1 tsp	0	Tr	Tr	Tr	Tr	Tr
Dried, ground	1 tsp	5	1	Tr	1	Tr	Tr
Pam, non-stick cooking spray	...	...	.	.	.	.	.
⅓ second spray	1 spray	0	0	0	0	0	0
Pam, Baking, ⅓ second spray	1 spray	0	0	0	0	0	0
Pancake, 4″ dia	...	...	.	.	.	.	.
Frozen	1	90	16	1	15	2	2
Regular, from mix	1	80	11	Tr	11	3	3
Whole wheat, from mix	1	90	13	1	12	4	3
Kellogg's Eggo Buttermilk Pancake	1	90	15	Tr	15	2	3
Pancake Syrup – see Syrup	...	...	.	.	.	.	.
Papaya	...	...	.	.	.	.	.
Fresh, peeled, 5″ long × 3″ dia	1	120	30	6	24	2	Tr
Fresh, peeled, cubed	1 cup	60	14	3	11	Tr	Tr
Paprika, dried powder	1 tsp	5	1	Tr	1	Tr	Tr
Parsley	...	...	.	.	.	.	.
Dried, leaves	1 Tbsp	0	Tr	Tr	Tr	Tr	Tr
Freeze-dried, leaves	1 Tbsp	0	Tr	Tr	Tr	Tr	Tr
Fresh, whole sprigs	10	0	Tr	Tr	Tr	Tr	Tr
Fresh, chopped	¼ cup	5	Tr	Tr	Tr	Tr	Tr
Parsnip	...	...	.	.	.	.	.
Sliced, cooked	½ cup	60	13	3	10	1	Tr
Whole, 9″ long, cooked	1	110	27	6	21	2	Tr
Passion Fruit, raw, avg size	1	15	4	2	2	Tr	Tr

	SERVING SIZE	CALORIES	TOTAL CARBS (g)	FIBER (g)	NET CARBS (g)	PROTEIN (g)	FAT (g)
Pasta	...	...	·	·	·	·	·
Spaghetti	...	...	·	·	·	·	·
Plain, cooked	1 cup	220	43	3	40	8	1
Plain, dry	2 oz	210	43	2	41	7	Tr
Spinach, dry	2 oz	210	43	6	37	8	Tr
Whole wheat, cooked	1 cup	170	37	6	31	8	Tr
Small shells, cooked	1 cup	180	36	2	34	7	1
Spiral shaped, cooked	1 cup	210	41	2	39	8	1
Rice pasta, cooked	1 cup	250	43	5	38	5	6
Tortellini, cheese-filled	¾ cup	250	38	2	36	11	6
Pastrami	...	...	·	·	·	·	·
Regular, beef	2 oz	80	0	0	0	12	3
Regular, beef 98% fat free	2 oz	50	Tr	0	Tr	11	Tr
Turkey	2 oz	80	1	Tr	1	9	4
Pastry – see Danish Pastry &	...	...	·	·	·	·	·
specific listings	...	...	·	·	·	·	·
Pastry Filling - see specific listing	...	...	·	·	·	·	·
Peach	...	...	·	·	·	·	·
Fresh, whole, med, 2⅔" dia	1	60	14	2	12	1	Tr
Fresh, sliced	1 cup	60	15	2	13	1	Tr
Canned, in heavy syrup	1 cup	190	52	3	49	1	Tr
Canned, in heavy syrup	1 half	70	20	1	19	Tr	Tr
Canned, in light syrup	1 cup	140	37	3	34	1	Tr

	SERVING SIZE	CALORIES	TOTAL CARBS (g)	FIBER (g)	NET CARBS (g)	PROTEIN (g)	FAT (g)
Canned, in light syrup	1 half	50	14	1	13	Tr	Tr
Canned, in juice	1 cup	110	29	3	26	2	Tr
Canned, in juice	1 half	45	11	1	10	Tr	Tr
Dried, halves	3	90	24	3	21	1	Tr
Frozen, sweetened slices, thawed	1 cup	240	60	5	55	2	Tr
Peanut – see Nuts	...	...	.	.	.	.	.
Peanut Butter	...	...	.	.	.	.	.
Regular, smooth	2 Tbsp	190	6	2	4	8	16
Regular, chunky	2 Tbsp	190	7	3	4	8	16
Reduced fat, smooth	2 Tbsp	170	11	2	9	8	11
Pear	...	...	.	.	.	.	.
Fresh, whole, med	1	100	28	6	22	Tr	Tr
Fresh, sliced	1 cup	80	22	4	18	Tr	Tr
Fresh, Asian, 3" dia	1	120	29	10	19	1	Tr
Canned, in heavy syrup	1 cup	200	51	4	47	Tr	Tr
Canned, in heavy syrup	1 half	60	15	1	14	Tr	Tr
Canned, in light syrup	1 cup	140	38	4	34	Tr	Tr
Canned, in light syrup	1 half	45	12	1	11	Tr	Tr
Canned, in juice	1 cup	120	32	4	28	Tr	Tr
Canned, in juice	1 half	40	10	1	9	Tr	Tr
Peas (cooked w/o fats)	...	...	.	.	.	.	.
Green peas, canned	½ cup	60	11	4	7	4	Tr
Green peas, baby, canned	½ cup	60	10	4	6	4	Tr
Green peas, fresh	½ cup	70	13	4	9	4	Tr
Green peas, frozen	½ cup	60	11	4	7	4	Tr

	SERVING SIZE	CALORIES	TOTAL CARBS (g)	FIBER (g)	NET CARBS (g)	PROTEIN (g)	FAT (g)
Lentils	½ cup	120	20	8	12	9	Tr
Pigeon peas (red gram)	½ cup	100	20	6	14	6	Tr
Split peas	½ cup	120	21	8	13	8	Tr
Pea Pods	. . .	. . .	.	.	.	.	.
Fresh, raw, whole	1 cup	25	5	2	3	2	Tr
Fresh, raw, chopped	½ cup	20	4	1	3	1	Tr
Fresh, cooked	½ cup	35	6	2	4	3	Tr
Frozen, cooked	½ cup	40	7	3	4	3	Tr
Peas and Carrots	. . .	. . .	.	.	.	.	.
Canned	½ cup	50	11	3	8	3	Tr
Frozen, cooked	½ cup	40	8	3	5	3	Tr
Peas and Onions	. . .	. . .	.	.	.	.	.
Canned	½ cup	30	5	1	4	2	Tr
Frozen, cooked	½ cup	40	8	2	6	2	Tr
Pecan Pie	1 slice	540	79	3	76	6	22
Pecans	. . .	. . .	.	.	.	.	.
Chopped	½ cup	380	8	5	3	5	39
Halves, about 20	1 oz	200	4	3	1	3	20
Pepper, dried powder or granules	. . .	. . .	.	.	.	.	.
Black	1 tsp	5	1	Tr	1	Tr	Tr
Cayenne or red	1 tsp	5	1	Tr	1	Tr	Tr
White	1 tsp	5	2	Tr	2	Tr	Tr
Pepperoni, 14 slices	1 oz	140	0	0	0	6	12
Peppers	. . .	. . .	.	.	.	.	.
Chili Peppers, hot, red or green	. . .	. . .	.	.	.	.	.
fresh, whole	1	20	4	Tr	4	Tr	Tr
fresh, chopped	½ cup	30	7	1	6	2	Tr
canned, chopped	½ cup	15	4	Tr	4	Tr	Tr

	SERVING SIZE	CALORIES	TOTAL CARBS (g)	FIBER (g)	NET CARBS (g)	PROTEIN (g)	FAT (g)
Green, sweet, raw	...	...	.	.	.	.	.
whole, lg, 3" dia	1	35	8	3	5	1	Tr
sliced	1 cup	20	4	2	2	Tr	Tr
chopped	1 cup	30	7	3	4	1	Tr
canned, chopped	1 cup	25	6	2	4	1	Tr
Jalapeno	...	...	.	.	.	.	.
fresh, whole	1	0	Tr	Tr	Tr	Tr	Tr
fresh, sliced	1 cup	25	5	3	2	1	Tr
canned, sliced	1 cup	30	5	3	2	Tr	Tr
Pasilla, dried, whole	1	25	4	2	2	Tr	Tr
Red, sweet, raw	...	...	.	.	.	.	.
whole, lg, 3" dia	1	50	10	3	7	2	Tr
sliced	1 cup	30	6	2	4	Tr	Tr
chopped	1 cup	45	9	3	6	2	Tr
canned, halves	1 cup	25	6	2	4	1	Tr
Red or Green, sweet	...	...	.	.	.	.	.
chopped, cooked	1 cup	40	9	2	7	1	Tr
Yellow, sweet, raw	...	...	.	.	.	.	.
whole, lg, 3" dia	1	50	12	2	10	2	Tr
strips	10	15	3	Tr	3	Tr	Tr
Persimmon	...	...	.	.	.	.	.
native, fresh, whole	1	30	8	2	6	Tr	Tr
Japanese, fresh, whole	1	120	31	6	25	Tr	Tr
Pickle	...	...	.	.	.	.	.
Bread & Butter, slices	6	40	10	Tr	10	Tr	Tr
Dill, whole, 4" long	1	15	4	2	2	Tr	Tr
Dill, spear	1	0	Tr	Tr	Tr	Tr	Tr
Sour, whole, 4" long	1	15	3	2	1	Tr	Tr
Sour, spear	1	0	Tr	Tr	Tr	Tr	Tr

	SERVING SIZE	CALORIES	TOTAL CARBS (g)	FIBER (g)	NET CARBS (g)	PROTEIN (g)	FAT (g)
Sweet Gherkin, whole, lg, 3″ long	1	30	7	Tr	7	Tr	Tr
Sweet Gherkin, whole, sm, 2⅛″ long	1	5	1	Tr	1	Tr	Tr
Pickle Relish	1 Tbsp	20	5	Tr	5	Tr	Tr
packet	1	15	4	Tr	4	Tr	Tr
Pie (⅛ of 9″ pie unless noted)	. . .	. . .	.	.	.	.	.
Apple pie	1 slice	300	43	2	41	2	14
Apple pie, Dutch	1 slice	400	61	2	59	3	16
Blueberry pie	1 slice	290	44	1	43	2	13
Boston Cream Pie–see Cake	. . .	. . .	.	.	.	.	.
Cherry pie	1 slice	330	50	1	49	3	14
Cherry, fried pie, 5″ × 3¾″	1	400	55	3	52	4	21
Chocolate Cream pie, ⅙ of 8″ pie	1 slice	340	38	2	36	3	22
Coconut Custard pie, ⅙ of 8″ pie	1 slice	270	31	2	29	6	14
Coconut Creme Pie, ⅙ of 7″ pie	1 slice	190	24	Tr	24	1	11
Lemon Meringue pie, ⅙ of 8″ pie	1 slice	300	53	1	52	2	10
Lemon, fried pie, 5″ × 3¾″	1	400	55	3	52	4	21
Peach pie, ⅙ of 8″ pie	1 slice	260	39	Tr	39	2	12
Pecan pie	1 slice	540	79	3	76	6	22
Pumpkin pie	1 slice	320	46	2	44	5	13

	SERVING SIZE	CALORIES	TOTAL CARBS (g)	FIBER (g)	NET CARBS (g)	PROTEIN (g)	FAT (g)
Pie Crust, 9″ dia	...	...	.	.	.	.	.
Regular, from recipe	1 crust	950	86	3	83	12	62
Regular, from frozen	1 crust	780	87	5	82	10	44
Regular, from dry mix	1 crust	800	81	3	78	11	49
Graham cracker crust, ready crust	1 crust	920	118	4	114	9	45
Graham cracker, from recipe	1 crust	1180	156	4	152	10	60
Chocolate wafer, from recipe	1 crust	1130	121	3	118	11	69
Chocolate wafer, ready crust	1 crust	880	117	5	112	11	41
Vanilla wafer, from recipe	1 crust	940	88	Tr	88	7	64
Pilaf – see Rice Pilaf	...	...	.	.	.	.	.
Pineapple	...	...	.	.	.	.	.
Fresh, chunks	1 cup	80	22	2	20	Tr	Tr
Fresh, slice ½″ dia	1	30	7	Tr	7	Tr	Tr
Canned, in heavy syrup,	...	...	.	.	.	.	.
chunks or crushed	1 cup	200	51	2	49	Tr	Tr
slice, 3″ dia	1	40	10	Tr	10	Tr	Tr
Canned, in light syrup	...	...	.	.	.	.	.
chunks or crushed	1 cup	130	34	2	32	Tr	Tr
slice, 3″ dia	1	25	7	Tr	7	Tr	Tr
Canned, in juice,	...	...	.	.	.	.	.
chunks or crushed	1 cup	150	39	2	37	1	Tr
slice, 3″ dia	1	30	7	Tr	7	Tr	Tr
Frozen, chunks, sweetened	1 cup	210	54	3	51	Tr	Tr

	SERVING SIZE	CALORIES	TOTAL CARBS (g)	FIBER (g)	NET CARBS (g)	PROTEIN (g)	FAT (g)
PIZZA (Listings for an avg size	...	...	.	.	.	.	.
slice, ⅛ of 14" pizza)	...	...	.	.	.	.	.
Thin Crust, Cheese	1 slice	190	17	1	16	9	10
Regular Crust	...	...	.	.	.	.	.
Cheese	1 slice	270	34	2	32	12	10
Pepperoni & Cheese	1 slice	300	34	2	32	13	12
Meat & Vegetables	1 slice	330	35	3	32	15	15
Thick Crust	...	...	.	.	.	.	.
Cheese	1 slice	290	33	2	31	13	12
Frozen	...	...	.	.	.	.	.
Healthy Choice, Cheese	1 pizza	350	55	5	50	20	5
Healthy Choice, Pepperoni	1 pizza	350	54	5	49	22	5
Healthy Choice, Supreme	1 pizza	340	53	4	49	20	4
Lean Cuisine, Deluxe Pizza	1 pizza	350	50	3	47	19	8
Lean Cuisine, Pepperoni Pizza	1 pizza	370	53	4	49	20	9
Lean Cuisine, Margherita Pizza	1 pizza	340	50	3	47	14	9
Smart Ones, Four Cheese Pizza	1 pizza	370	57	4	53	18	7
Smart Ones, Pepperoni Pizza	1 pizza	390	58	4	54	20	8
Plantain, without peel	...	...	.	.	.	.	.
Fresh, whole, medium size	1	220	57	4	53	2	Tr

	SERVING SIZE	CALORIES	TOTAL CARBS (g)	FIBER (g)	NET CARBS (g)	PROTEIN (g)	FAT (g)
Cooked, mashed	1 cup	230	62	5	57	2	Tr
Cooked, slices	1 cup	180	48	4	44	1	Tr
Plum	...	...	.	.	.	.	.
Fresh, whole, med, 2⅛" dia	1	30	8	Tr	8	Tr	Tr
Fresh, sliced	1 cup	80	19	2	17	1	Tr
Canned, in heavy syrup	1 cup	230	60	2	58	Tr	Tr
Canned, in light syrup	1 cup	160	41	2	39	Tr	Tr
Canned, in juice	1 cup	150	38	2	36	1	Tr
Dried-see Prunes	...	...	.	.	.	.	.
Pomegranate	...	...	.	.	.	.	.
Fresh, whole, 4" dia	1	230	53	11	42	5	3
Fresh, seeds	½ cup	70	16	4	12	2	1
Pop Tart – see Toaster Pastry	...	...	.	.	.	.	.
Popcorn	...	...	.	.	.	.	.
Air popped	1 cup	30	6	1	5	1	Tr
Caramel coated w/ peanuts	⅔ cup	110	23	1	22	2	2
Cheese flavored	1 cup	60	6	1	5	1	4
Microwave, butter flavor	1 cup	40	5	Tr	5	Tr	2
Microwave, butter, reduced fat	1 cup	30	6	1	5	1	Tr
Microwave, 94% fat free	1 cup	30	6	1	5	Tr	Tr
Popped in oil	1 cup	60	6	1	5	Tr	3
Popcorn Cake, plain	1	40	8	Tr	8	Tr	Tr
Popsicle – see Frozen Dessert	...	...	.	.	.	.	.

	SERVING SIZE	CALORIES	TOTAL CARBS (g)	FIBER (g)	NET CARBS (g)	PROTEIN (g)	FAT (g)
PORK	...	...	.	.	.	.	.
(Weights for meat w/o bones)	...	...	.	.	.	.	.
Bacon	...	...	.	.	.	.	.
regular	1 slice	45	Tr	0	Tr	3	3
Canadian	2 slices	90	Tr	0	Tr	11	4
Boston Butt, braised	...	...	.	.	.	.	.
lean & fat	3 oz	230	0	0	0	21	15
lean only	3 oz	200	0	0	0	23	11
Picnic Pork, roasted	...	...	.	.	.	.	.
lean & fat	3 oz	270	0	0	0	20	20
lean only	3 oz	190	0	0	0	23	11
Pork Chop, loin cut	...	...	.	.	.	.	.
broiled, lean & fat	3 oz	220	0	0	0	24	13
broiled, lean only	3 oz	180	0	0	0	25	9
pan fried, lean & fat	3 oz	230	0	0	0	22	15
pan fried, lean only	3 oz	190	0	0	0	24	10
Rib Roast, lean & fat	3 oz	210	0	0	0	23	13
lean only	3 oz	180	0	0	0	25	9
Ribs, country-style, roasted	...	...	.	.	.	.	.
lean & fat	3 oz	280	0	0	0	20	22
lean only	3 oz	210	0	0	0	23	13
Sausage	...	...	.	.	.	.	.
Oscar Mayer, pork sausage links	2	170	Tr	0	Tr	8	15
liver (braunschweiger), ¼" slice	1	60	Tr	0	Tr	3	5
liverwurst, ¼" slice	1	60	Tr	0	Tr	3	5

	SERVING SIZE	CALORIES	TOTAL CARBS (g)	FIBER (g)	NET CARBS (g)	PROTEIN (g)	FAT (g)
sausage, regular	2 oz	190	0	0	0	11	16
smoked, 4" link	1	210	Tr	0	Tr	8	19
Polish Kielbasa sausage	2 oz	190	Tr	0	Tr	8	16
Vienna sausage, 2" links	2	70	Tr	0	Tr	3	6
Shoulder, roasted, lean & fat	3 oz	250	0	0	0	20	18
lean only	3 oz	200	0	0	0	22	12
Spareribs, braised	3 oz	340	0	0	0	25	26
(Other Pork Products, see:	...	...	.	.	.	.	.
Bologna, Ham, Hot Dog,	...	...	.	.	.	.	.
Salami, & specific entrèes)	...	...	.	.	.	.	.
Pork Rinds	1 oz	150	0	0	0	17	9
Pot Pie, frozen, heated	...	...	.	.	.	.	.
Beef Pot Pie	1 pie	590	59	2	57	19	31
Chicken Pot Pie	1 pie	500	54	3	51	14	25
Turkey Pot Pie	1 pie	700	70	4	66	26	35
Banquet	...	...	.	.	.	.	.
Beef Pot Pie	1 pie	450	36	2	34	14	27
Chicken Pot Pie	1 pie	370	34	2	32	10	21
Chicken w/ Broccoli Pot Pie	1 pie	350	32	2	30	10	20
Turkey Pot Pie	1 pie	390	36	2	34	10	21
Marie Callender's	...	...	.	.	.	.	.
Beef Pot Pie	1 cup	540	46	3	43	16	32
Cheesy Chicken Pot Pie	1 cup	600	46	3	43	17	37
Chicken Pot Pie	1 cup	530	48	3	45	14	31

	SERVING SIZE	CALORIES	TOTAL CARBS (g)	FIBER (g)	NET CARBS (g)	PROTEIN (g)	FAT (g)
Creamy Mushroom & Chicken Pot Pie	1 cup	560	45	3	42	15	35
Creamy Parmesan Chicken Pot Pie	1 cup	530	43	2	41	17	32
Honey Roasted Chicken Pot Pie	1 cup	530	47	3	44	16	30
Turkey Pot Pie	1 cup	530	45	4	41	15	32
Stouffer's	...	...	.	.	.	.	.
White Meat Chicken Pot Pie	1 pie	660	62	2	60	19	37
White Meat Turkey Pot Pie	1 pie	710	61	2	59	23	41
Pot Roast – see Frozen Dinner	...	...	.	.	.	.	.
POTATO	...	...	.	.	.	.	.
(also see Sweet Potatoes)	...	...	.	.	.	.	.
Au Gratin Potatoes	1 cup	320	28	4	24	12	19
Baked potato, med	...	...	.	.	.	.	.
whole potato w/ skin	1	160	37	4	33	4	Tr
whole potato w/o skin	1	150	34	2	32	3	Tr
skin only	1	120	27	5	22	3	Tr
peeled, whole potato	1	120	27	2	25	3	Tr
peeled, diced	½ cup	70	16	1	15	2	Tr
French Fries	...	...	.	.	.	.	.
Frozen, heated	...	...	.	.	.	.	.
thin shoestring	10 fries	40	7	Tr	7	Tr	1
regular or crinkle cut	10 fries	120	19	2	17	2	4

	SERVING SIZE	CALORIES	TOTAL CARBS (g)	FIBER (g)	NET CARBS (g)	PROTEIN (g)	FAT (g)
steak fries	10 fries	200	36	4	32	3	5
Hash Browns, frozen, heated, patty, 3" × 1½"	1	60	8	Tr	8	Tr	3
Hash Browned potatoes	1 cup	410	55	5	50	5	20
Mashed, w/milk & butter	1 cup	240	35	3	32	4	9
Mashed, dehydrated, as prep w/milk & butter	1 cup	230	30	5	25	4	10
Scalloped potatoes	1 cup	220	26	5	21	7	9
Tater Tots/potato puffs, frozen, heated	10	150	22	2	20	2	7
Potato Chips	...	...	.	.	.	.	.
(about 14 chips, unless noted)	...	...	.	.	.	.	.
Plain, regular	1 oz	150	15	1	14	2	10
Barbecue flavor	1 oz	140	15	1	14	2	9
Cheese flavor	1 oz	140	16	2	14	2	8
Fat free chips	1 oz	80	18	2	16	2	Tr
Pringles, regular (about 16 crisps)	1 oz	150	15	1	14	1	9
Reduced fat chips	1 oz	130	19	2	17	2	6
Ruffles, original	1 oz	160	14	1	13	2	10
Ruffles, reduced fat	1 oz	140	18	1	17	2	7
Sour cream & onion flavor	1 oz	150	15	2	13	2	10
Potato Pancakes, 2 ¾" dia	1	60	6	Tr	6	1	3

	SERVING SIZE	CALORIES	TOTAL CARBS (g)	FIBER (g)	NET CARBS (g)	PROTEIN (g)	FAT (g)
Potato Salad	1 cup	360	28	3	25	7	21
Potato Sticks, fried, crunchy	½ cup	90	10	Tr	10	1	6
Preserves	. . .	. . .	.	.	.	.	.
All flavors, regular	1 Tbsp	60	14	Tr	14	Tr	Tr
Restaurant size packet	½ oz	40	10	Tr	10	Tr	Tr
Pretzels	. . .	. . .	.	.	.	.	.
Twists	10	230	48	2	46	6	2
Soft, twisted, med	1	390	80	2	78	9	4
Prickly pear	. . .	. . .	.	.	.	.	.
Fresh, whole	1	40	10	4	6	Tr	Tr
Fresh, sliced	1 cup	60	14	5	9	1	Tr
Prosciutto, *Boarshead*	1 oz	60	0	0	0	8	3
Prunes, dried, pitted	. . .	. . .	.	.	.	.	.
Uncooked, unsweetened	5 prunes	110	30	3	27	1	Tr
Stewed, unsweetened	1 cup	270	70	8	62	2	Tr
Pudding	. . .	. . .	. . .	. . .	. . .	. . .	. . .
Banana, regular	4 oz	130	21	0	21	3	3
instant	4 oz	130	22	0	22	3	3
Chocolate, regular	½ cup	170	28	1	27	5	5
instant	½ cup	160	28	2	26	5	5
fat free	½ cup	110	24	Tr	24	2	Tr
Coconut Cream, regular	½ cup	160	25	Tr	25	4	5
instant	½ cup	170	28	Tr	28	4	5
Lemon, instant	½ cup	170	30	0	30	4	4
Rice pudding, regular	4 oz	130	22	1	21	4	3

	SERVING SIZE	CALORIES	TOTAL CARBS (g)	FIBER (g)	NET CARBS (g)	PROTEIN (g)	FAT (g)
Tapioca, regular	4 oz	140	24	0	24	2	4
fat free	4 oz	110	24	0	24	2	Tr
Vanilla, regular	½ cup	160	26	Tr	26	4	4
instant	½ cup	160	28	0	28	4	4
fat free	4 oz	100	23	0	23	2	0
Puff Pastry, frozen, baked	1 sheet	1370	112	4	108	18	94
Individual shell	1	220	18	Tr	18	3	15
Pumpkin	. . .	. . .	.	.	.	.	.
Fresh, cooked, mashed	1 cup	50	12	3	9	2	Tr
Canned	1 cup	80	20	7	13	3	Tr
Pumpkin Pie Mix, canned	1 cup	280	71	22	49	3	Tr
Pumpkin Pie Spice	1 tsp	5	1	Tr	1	Tr	Tr
Quesadilla – see individual restaurant listings	. . .	. . .	.	.	.	.	.
Radish, fresh, raw, med	5	0	Tr	Tr	Tr	Tr	Tr
Sliced	1 cup	20	4	2	2	Tr	Tr
Raisin	. . .	. . .	.	.	.	.	.
Golden, not packed	1 cup	440	115	6	109	5	Tr
Regular, not packed	1 cup	430	115	5	110	5	Tr
small box	1½ oz	130	34	2	32	1	Tr
miniature box	½ oz	40	11	Tr	11	Tr	Tr
Raisin Bran – see Cereal	. . .	. . .	.	.	.	.	.
Raspberries	. . .	. . .	.	.	.	.	.
Fresh	1 cup	60	15	8	7	2	Tr
Frozen, sweetened, unthawed	1 cup	260	65	11	54	2	Tr

	SERVING SIZE	CALORIES	TOTAL CARBS (g)	FIBER (g)	NET CARBS (g)	PROTEIN (g)	FAT (g)
Ravioli, *Chef Boyardee*	...	...	·	·	·	·	·
Beef	1 cup	220	33	1	32	8	7
Mini ravioli, beef	1 cup	230	31	3	28	8	8
Relish – see Pickle Relish or	...	...	·	·	·	·	·
specific listing	...	...	·	·	·	·	·
Rhubarb	...	...	·	·	·	·	·
Fresh, diced	1 cup	25	6	2	4	1	Tr
Frozen, cooked, sweetened	1 cup	280	75	5	70	Tr	Tr
RICE	...	...	·	·	·	·	·
Plain Rice Dishes	...	...	·	·	·	·	·
Brown rice, med grain, cooked	1 cup	220	46	4	42	5	2
Brown rice, long grain, cooked	1 cup	220	45	4	41	5	2
White rice, med grain, cooked	1 cup	240	53	Tr	53	4	Tr
White rice, long grain, cooked	1 cup	210	45	Tr	45	4	Tr
White rice, parboiled, cooked	1 cup	190	42	1	41	5	Tr
White rice, instant, as prep	1 cup	190	41	1	40	4	Tr
White rice, glutinous, cooked	1 cup	170	37	2	35	4	Tr
Wild rice, cooked	1 cup	170	35	3	32	7	Tr
Rice Cake, brown rice	1	35	7	Tr	7	Tr	Tr
Rice Krispies Treat	1 bar	150	30	Tr	30	1	3
Roast Beef – see Beef	...	...	·	·	·	·	·

	SERVING SIZE	CALORIES	TOTAL CARBS (g)	FIBER (g)	NET CARBS (g)	PROTEIN (g)	FAT (g)
Rolls – see Bread	...	...	.	.	.	.	.
Rosemary	...	...	.	.	.	.	.
Dried spice	1 tsp	0	Tr	Tr	Tr	Tr	Tr
Fresh, chopped	1 tsp	0	Tr	Tr	Tr	Tr	Tr
Rutabaga	...	...	.	.	.	.	.
Cubed, cooked	1 cup	70	15	3	12	2	Tr
Mashed, cooked	1 cup	90	21	4	17	3	Tr
Saccharin sweetener	1 pkt	0	Tr	0	Tr	Tr	0
Sage, dried, ground	1 tsp	0	Tr	Tr	Tr	Tr	Tr
SALAD DRESSING	...	...	.	.	.	.	.
Blue cheese, regular	1 Tbsp	70	Tr	Tr	Tr	Tr	8
Blue cheese, low calorie	1 Tbsp	15	Tr	0	Tr	Tr	1
Blue cheese, fat free	1 Tbsp	20	4	Tr	4	Tr	Tr
Buttermilk, lite	1 Tbsp	30	3	Tr	3	Tr	2
Caesar, regular	1 Tbsp	80	Tr	Tr	Tr	Tr	9
Caesar, low calorie	1 Tbsp	15	3	0	3	Tr	Tr
French, regular	1 Tbsp	70	3	0	3	Tr	7
French, low calorie	1 Tbsp	30	4	0	4	Tr	2
French, low fat	1 Tbsp	35	5	Tr	5	Tr	2
French, fat free	1 Tbsp	20	5	Tr	5	Tr	Tr
Honey mustard, low calorie	1 Tbsp	60	9	Tr	9	Tr	3
Italian, regular	1 Tbsp	40	2	0	2	Tr	4
Italian, low calorie	1 Tbsp	30	Tr	0	Tr	Tr	3
Italian, low fat	1 Tbsp	10	Tr	0	Tr	Tr	Tr
Italian, fat free	1 Tbsp	5	1	Tr	1	Tr	Tr
Mayonnaise, regular	1 Tbsp	100	Tr	0	Tr	Tr	11
Mayonnaise, light	1 Tbsp	50	1	0	1	Tr	5
Mayonnaise, fat free	1 Tbsp	15	3	Tr	3	Tr	Tr

	SERVING SIZE	CALORIES	TOTAL CARBS (g)	FIBER (g)	NET CARBS (g)	PROTEIN (g)	FAT (g)
Ranch, regular	1 Tbsp	70	1	Tr	1	Tr	8
Ranch, low fat	1 Tbsp	30	3	Tr	3	Tr	2
Ranch, fat free	1 Tbsp	15	4	0	4	Tr	Tr
Russian, regular	1 Tbsp	50	5	Tr	5	Tr	4
Russian, low calorie	1 Tbsp	25	4	0	4	Tr	Tr
Thousand island, regular	1 Tbsp	60	2	Tr	2	Tr	6
Thousand island, low fat	1 Tbsp	30	4	Tr	4	Tr	2
Thousand island, fat free	1 Tbsp	20	5	Tr	5	Tr	Tr
Salami	. . .	. . .	.	.	.	.	.
Turkey, cooked	1 oz	45	Tr	0	Tr	5	3
Beef, cooked	1 oz	70	Tr	0	Tr	4	6
Pork, hard or dry	1 oz	110	Tr	0	Tr	6	9
sliced, 3" × ⅟₁₆" slices	2	80	Tr	0	Tr	5	7
Pork, Italian	1 oz	120	Tr	0	Tr	6	10
Salsa	1 Tbsp	0	1	Tr	1	Tr	Tr
Salt, table	. . .	. . .	.	.	.	.	.
Regular	½ tsp	0	0	0	0	0	0
Sandwich Meat – see Lunch Meat	. . .	. . .	.	.	.	.	.
Sandwich Spread, pork, beef	1 Tbsp	35	2	0	2	1	3
Poultry	1 Tbsp	25	Tr	0	Tr	2	2
SAUCE	. . .	. . .	.	.	.	.	.
A1 Steak Sauce	1 Tbsp	30	8	Tr	8	Tr	0
Barbecue sauce	1 Tbsp	25	6	Tr	6	0	Tr
Catsup	1 Tbsp	15	4	0	4	Tr	Tr
Cheese sauce	¼ cup	110	4	Tr	4	4	8

	SERVING SIZE	CALORIES	TOTAL CARBS (g)	FIBER (g)	NET CARBS (g)	PROTEIN (g)	FAT (g)
Chili sauce	¼ cup	70	14	4	10	2	Tr
Hoison sauce	1 Tbsp	35	7	Tr	7	Tr	Tr
Horseradish, prepared	1 tsp	0	Tr	Tr	Tr	Tr	Tr
Hot sauce	1 tsp	0	Tr	0	Tr	Tr	Tr
Marinara sauce	½ cup	110	18	3	15	2	3
Mayonnaise, regular	1 Tbsp	100	Tr	0	Tr	Tr	11
Mayonnaise, light	1 Tbsp	50	1	0	1	Tr	5
Mayonnaise, fat free	1 Tbsp	15	3	Tr	3	Tr	Tr
Mustard, regular	1 tsp	0	Tr	Tr	Tr	Tr	Tr
Oyster sauce	1 Tbsp	10	2	Tr	2	Tr	Tr
Pasta sauce	½ cup	110	18	3	15	2	3
Pepper sauce, hot	1 tsp	0	Tr	0	Tr	Tr	Tr
Pickle Relish	1 Tbsp	20	5	Tr	5	Tr	Tr
Pizza sauce	¼ cup	35	6	1	5	1	Tr
Plum sauce	1 Tbsp	35	8	Tr	8	Tr	Tr
Salsa	1 Tbsp	0	1	Tr	1	Tr	Tr
Sofrito	½ cup	240	6	2	4	13	19
Soy sauce	1 Tbsp	10	1	Tr	1	1	Tr
Spaghetti sauce	½ cup	110	18	3	15	2	3
Sweet & Sour Sauce	1 Tbsp	15	3	Tr	3	Tr	Tr
Tabasco sauce	1 tsp	0	Tr	0	Tr	Tr	Tr
Tamari Sauce	1 Tbsp	10	1	Tr	1	2	Tr
Teriyaki sauce	1 Tbsp	15	3	0	3	1	0
Tomato sauce	½ cup	30	7	2	5	2	Tr
White sauce	½ cup	180	12	Tr	12	5	13
Worcestershire sauce	1 Tbsp	15	3	0	3	0	0
Sauerkraut	1 cup	45	10	7	3	2	Tr

	SERVING SIZE	CALORIES	TOTAL CARBS (g)	FIBER (g)	NET CARBS (g)	PROTEIN (g)	FAT (g)
Sausage (see also, Pork)	...	...	.	.	.	.	.
Beef sausage	2 oz	190	Tr	0	Tr	10	16
Beef sausage, cured, smoked	1 oz	90	Tr	0	Tr	4	8
Beef & Pork sausage	2 oz	220	2	0	2	8	20
Beef & Pork sausage, smoked	2 oz	180	1	0	1	7	16
Blood sausage	2 oz	210	Tr	0	Tr	8	19
Chicken & Beef, smoked	2 oz	170	0	0	0	10	13
Lowfat sausage, beef, pork, & turkey	2 oz	60	6	Tr	6	5	1
Sweet Italian sausage, 3 oz link	1	130	2	0	2	14	7
Turkey sausage	2 oz	110	0	0	0	13	6
Turkey & Pork sausage	2 oz	170	Tr	0	Tr	13	13
Polish sausage, Kielbasa	2 oz	130	2	0	2	7	10
Vienna sausage, 2" links	2 links	70	Tr	0	Tr	3	6
Scallop – see Fish/ Seafood	...	...	.	.	.	.	.
Seafood – see Fish/ Seafood	...	...	.	.	.	.	.
Seasoning – see specific listings	...	...	.	.	.	.	.
Poultry	1 tsp	5	Tr	Tr	Tr	Tr	Tr
Seaweed	...	...	.	.	.	.	.
Agar, raw	2 Tbsp	0	Tr	Tr	Tr	Tr	0
Agar, dried	¼ oz	20	6	Tr	6	Tr	Tr
Kelp, raw	2 Tbsp	0	Tr	Tr	Tr	Tr	Tr

	SERVING SIZE	CALORIES	TOTAL CARBS (g)	FIBER (g)	NET CARBS (g)	PROTEIN (g)	FAT (g)
Spirulina, dried	1 Tbsp	20	2	Tr	2	4	Tr
Wakame, raw	2 Tbsp	5	Tr	Tr	Tr	Tr	Tr
Seeds	...	...	.	.	.	.	.
Flaxseed, whole	1 Tbsp	60	3	3	0	2	4
Flaxseed, ground	1 Tbsp	35	2	2	0	1	3
Pumpkin seeds, kernels, roasted	1 oz	150	4	1	3	9	12
Sesame seeds, plain	1 Tbsp	50	2	1	1	2	5
Sesame seeds, toasted	1 oz	160	7	4	3	5	14
Sunflower seeds, dry roasted	1 oz	170	7	3	4	6	14
(Also see specific listings)	...	...	.	.	.	.	.
Shallot, raw, chopped	1 Tbsp	5	2	Tr	2	Tr	Tr
Freeze-dried	1 Tbsp	0	Tr	Tr	Tr	Tr	0
Shark – see Fish	...	...	.	.	.	.	.
Sherbet, Orange	½ cup	110	23	1	22	Tr	2
Shortening, regular cottonseed &	1 cup	1810	0	0	0	0	205
soybean blend	1 Tbsp	110	0	0	0	0	13
Shrimp – see Fish/ Seafood	...	...	.	.	.	.	.
& specific entrèes	...	...	.	.	.	.	.
Sirloin Steak – see Beef	...	...	.	.	.	.	.
Snack Mix, *Chex Mix*	¾ cup	120	18	2	16	3	5
Oriental mix, rice-based	1 oz	140	15	4	11	5	7
SOUP (as prep)	...	...	.	.	.	.	.
Bouillon cube, chicken	1	10	Tr	0	Tr	Tr	Tr

	SERVING SIZE	CALORIES	TOTAL CARBS (g)	FIBER (g)	NET CARBS (g)	PROTEIN (g)	FAT (g)
Bouillon cube, low sodium	1	15	2	0	2	Tr	Tr
Bouillon cube, beef	1	10	Tr	0	Tr	Tr	Tr
Broth, beef	1 cup	15	Tr	0	Tr	3	Tr
Broth, chicken	1 cup	10	Tr	0	Tr	Tr	Tr
Broth, chicken, low sodium	1 cup	40	3	0	3	5	1
Broth, beef consommè, as prep	1 cup	30	2	0	2	5	0
Bean w/ Ham soup	1 cup	230	27	11	16	13	9
Bean w/ Pork soup	1 cup	170	22	8	14	8	6
Beef Noodle soup	1 cup	80	9	Tr	9	5	3
Beef Noodle Tomato soup	1 cup	140	21	2	19	4	4
Black Bean soup	1 cup	110	19	8	11	6	2
Cheese soup, prep w/ water	1 cup	160	11	1	10	5	11
Cheese soup, prep w/ milk	1 cup	230	16	1	15	10	15
Chicken Noodle soup, canned	1 cup	60	7	Tr	7	3	2
Chicken Noodle soup, dry mix, as prep	1 cup	60	9	Tr	9	2	1
Chicken Noodle soup, chunky	1 cup	90	10	1	9	8	2
Chicken & Rice soup	1 cup	60	7	Tr	7	4	2
Chicken & Rice soup, chunky	1 cup	130	13	1	12	12	3
Chicken & Vegetable, regular	1 cup	80	9	1	8	4	3
Chicken & Vegetable, chunky	1 cup	170	19	1	18	12	5

	SERVING SIZE	CALORIES	TOTAL CARBS (g)	FIBER (g)	NET CARBS (g)	PROTEIN (g)	FAT (g)
Clam Chowder, Manhattan	1 cup	80	12	2	10	2	2
Clam Chowder, Manhattan, chunky	1 cup	130	19	3	16	7	3
Clam Chowder, New England	...	...	.	.	.	.	.
prep w/ water	1 cup	90	13	Tr	13	4	3
prep w/ milk	1 cup	150	19	Tr	19	8	5
Cream of Asparagus	...	...	.	.	.	.	.
prep w/ water	1 cup	90	11	Tr	11	2	4
prep w/ milk	1 cup	160	16	Tr	16	6	8
Cream of Celery	...	...	.	.	.	.	.
prep w/ water	1 cup	90	9	Tr	9	2	6
prep w/ milk	1 cup	160	15	Tr	15	6	10
Cream of Chicken soup	...	...	.	.	.	.	.
prep w/ water	1 cup	120	9	Tr	9	3	7
prep w/ milk	1 cup	190	15	Tr	15	8	12
Cream of Mushroom soup	...	...	.	.	.	.	.
prep w/ water	1 cup	100	8	0	8	2	7
prep w/ milk	1 cup	170	14	0	14	6	10
Cream of Onion	...	...	.	.	.	.	.
prep w/ water	1 cup	110	13	1	12	3	5
prep w/ milk	1 cup	190	18	Tr	18	7	9
Cream of Potato	...	...	.	.	.	.	.
prep w/ water	1 cup	70	12	Tr	12	2	2
prep w/ milk	1 cup	150	17	Tr	17	6	7
Minestrone, regular	1 cup	80	11	1	10	4	3
Minestrone, chunky	1 cup	130	21	6	15	5	3
Miso, as prep	1 cup	20	3	Tr	3	1	Tr
Onion soup, canned	1 cup	60	8	Tr	8	4	2

	SERVING SIZE	CALORIES	TOTAL CARBS (g)	FIBER (g)	NET CARBS (g)	PROTEIN (g)	FAT (g)
Onion soup, dry mix, as prep	1 cup	30	6	Tr	6	Tr	Tr
Pea soup, green	1 cup	160	26	5	21	8	3
Ramen Beef Noodle soup	½ pkg	190	27	Tr	27	4	7
Ramen Chicken noodle soup	½ pkg	190	27	1	26	5	7
Split Pea w/ Ham	1 cup	190	28	2	26	10	4
Split Pea w/ Ham, chunky	1 cup	190	27	4	23	11	4
Tomato soup, prep w/ water	1 cup	70	16	2	14	2	Tr
Tomato soup, prep w/ milk	1 cup	140	22	2	20	6	3
Tomato bisque, prep w/ water	1 cup	120	24	Tr	24	2	3
Tomato bisque, prep w/ milk	1 cup	200	29	Tr	29	6	7
Tomato Rice	1 cup	120	21	2	19	2	3
Tomato Vegetable	1 cup	50	10	Tr	10	2	Tr
Turkey Vegetable	1 cup	70	9	Tr	9	3	3
Vegetable soup	1 cup	70	12	Tr	12	2	2
Vegetable Beef soup	1 cup	80	10	2	8	5	2
Sour cream	...	...	.	.	.	.	.
Regular	1 cup	440	7	0	7	5	45
Regular	1 Tbsp	25	Tr	0	Tr	Tr	2
Reduced fat	1 Tbsp	20	Tr	0	Tr	Tr	2
Fat free	1 Tbsp	12	3	0	3	Tr	0
Soy Burger	1 patty	120	10	3	7	11	4
Soybeans	...	...	.	.	.	.	.
green, cooked	½ cup	130	10	4	6	11	6
mature seeds, cooked	½ cup	150	9	5	4	14	8

	SERVING SIZE	CALORIES	TOTAL CARBS (g)	FIBER (g)	NET CARBS (g)	PROTEIN (g)	FAT (g)
Spaghetti – see Pasta	...	...	.	.	.	.	.
Spare Ribs – see Pork	...	...	.	.	.	.	.
Spice – see specific listings	...	...	.	.	.	.	.
Spinach	...	...	.	.	.	.	.
Fresh, raw	1 cup	5	1	Tr	1	Tr	Tr
Fresh, chopped, cooked	1 cup	40	7	4	3	5	Tr
Frozen, chopped, cooked	1 cup	70	9	7	2	8	2
Canned, cooked	1 cup	50	7	5	2	6	1
Spinach Soufflè	1 cup	230	8	1	7	11	18
Spread	...	...	.	.	.	.	.
Cheese Spread, pasteurized	1 oz	80	3	0	3	5	6
Cheese Spread, cream cheese base	1 Tbsp	45	Tr	0	Tr	1	4
Ham & Cheese Spread	1 Tbsp	40	Tr	0	Tr	2	3
Ham Salad Spread	1 Tbsp	30	2	0	2	1	2
Liverwurst Spread	1 Tbsp	40	Tr	Tr	Tr	2	4
Sandwich Spread, pork or beef	1 Tbsp	35	2	Tr	2	1	3
Sandwich Spread, poultry salad	1 Tbsp	26	Tr	0	Tr	2	2
(also see spreads in Margarine)	...	...	.	.	.	.	.
Squash	...	...	.	.	.	.	.
Acorn squash, baked, cubes	1 cup	120	30	9	21	2	Tr
Butternut squash, raw, cubed	1 cup	60	16	3	13	1	Tr

	SERVING SIZE	CALORIES	TOTAL CARBS (g)	FIBER (g)	NET CARBS (g)	PROTEIN (g)	FAT (g)
Hubbard squash, cooked, mashed	1 cup	70	15	7	8	4	Tr
Spaghetti squash, cooked	1 cup	40	10	2	8	1	Tr
Summer, raw, sliced	1 cup	20	4	1	3	1	Tr
Summer, cooked, slices	1 cup	35	8	3	5	2	Tr
Winter, baked, cubes	1 cup	80	18	6	12	2	Tr
Steak – see Beef	...	...	.	.	.		.
Steak Sauce, A1	1 Tbsp	30	8	Tr	8	Tr	0
Strawberries	...	...	.	.	.	.	.
Fresh, medium size, 1 ¼" dia	10	40	9	2	7	Tr	Tr
Fresh, sliced	1 cup	50	13	3	10	1	Tr
Frozen, unsweetened, thawed	1 cup	80	20	5	15	Tr	Tr
Frozen, sweetened, thawed	1 cup	250	66	5	61	1	Tr
Strawberry Topping – see Topping	...	...	.	.	.	.	.
Strudel, apple	1 piece	200	29	2	27	2	8
Stuffing	...	...	.	.	.	.	.
Bread, dry mix, as prep	½ cup	180	22	3	19	3	9
Cornbread dry mix, as prep	½ cup	180	22	3	19	3	9
Succotash	...	...	.	.	.	.	.
Canned	½ cup	80	18	3	15	3	Tr
Fresh, cooked	½ cup	110	23	4	19	5	Tr
Frozen, cooked	½ cup	80	17	4	13	4	Tr
Sugar	...	...	.	.	.	.	.
White, regular, granulated	...	...	.	.	.	.	.

	SERVING SIZE	CALORIES	TOTAL CARBS (g)	FIBER (g)	NET CARBS (g)	PROTEIN (g)	FAT (g)
One cup	1 cup	770	200	0	200	0	0
One tablespoon	1 Tbsp	50	13	0	13	0	0
One teaspoon	1 tsp	15	4	0	4	0	0
One cube	1	10	2	0	2	0	0
Restaurant size packet	1	10	3	0	3	0	0
White, Confectioner's, Powdered	...	...	.	.	.	.	.
Unsifted, one cup	1 cup	470	120	0	120	0	Tr
Sifted, one cup	1 cup	390	100	0	100	0	Tr
Unsifted, one tablespoon	1 Tbsp	30	8	0	8	0	Tr
Brown Sugar	...	...	.	.	.	.	.
Packed, one cup	1 cup	840	216	0	216	Tr	0
Packed, one tablespoon	1 Tbsp	50	14	0	14	Tr	0
Brownulated	1 Tbsp	35	9	0	9	Tr	0
Sugar Substitute	...	...	.	.	.	.	.
Aspartame sweetener	1 pkt	0	Tr	0	Tr	Tr	0
Saccharin sweetener	1 pkt	0	Tr	0	Tr	Tr	0
Sugar Twin	1 pkt	0	Tr	0	Tr	Tr	0
Sundae (small serving)	...	...	.	.	.	.	.
Caramel	1	300	49	0	49	7	9
Hot Fudge	1	280	48	0	48	6	9
Strawberry	1	270	45	0	45	6	8
Swedish Meatballs – see Frozen Dinner	...	...	.	.	.	.	.
Sweet 'N Low	1 pkt	0	Tr	0	Tr	Tr	0
Sweet Potato	...	...	.	.	.	.	.
Baked w/skin, whole, med, 5" × 2"	1	110	24	4	20	2	Tr

	SERVING SIZE	CALORIES	TOTAL CARBS (g)	FIBER (g)	NET CARBS (g)	PROTEIN (g)	FAT (g)
Cooked, mashed	½ cup	90	21	3	18	2	Tr
Candied, 2½″ × 2″ pieces	1 piece	150	29	3	26	Tr	3
Canned in syrup, drained	1 cup	210	50	6	44	3	Tr
Canned, mashed, vacuum pack	1 cup	230	54	5	49	4	Tr
Frozen, baked, cubes	1 cup	180	41	3	38	3	Tr
Sweet Potato Chips	1 oz	140	18	1	17	Tr	7
Sweet Roll – see specific listings	...	...	·	·	·	·	·
Syrup	...	...	·	·	·	·	·
Chocolate fudge, thick	2 Tbsp	130	24	1	23	2	3
Corn, light	1 Tbsp	60	17	0	17	0	Tr
Corn, dark	1 Tbsp	60	16	0	16	0	0
Grenadine	1 Tbsp	50	13	0	13	0	0
Malt	1 Tbsp	80	17	0	17	2	0
Maple	1 Tbsp	50	13	0	13	0	Tr
Molasses	1 Tbsp	60	15	0	15	0	Tr
Molasses	1 cup	980	252	0	252	0	Tr
Pancake Syrup/ Table Syrup	...	...	·	·	·	·	·
Regular	1 Tbsp	45	12	0	12	0	0
Light, reduced calorie	1 Tbsp	25	7	0	7	0	0
Taco – see individual restaurant listings	...	...	·	·	·	·	·
Taco Shell, med 5″ dia	1	60	8	Tr	8	Tr	3
Tahini, from toasted kernels	1 Tbsp	90	3	1	2	3	8
Tangerine, fresh, med, 2 ½″ dia	1	45	12	2	10	Tr	Tr

	SERVING SIZE	CALORIES	TOTAL CARBS (g)	FIBER (g)	NET CARBS (g)	PROTEIN (g)	FAT (g)
Tapioca, pearl, dry	1 cup	540	135	1	134	Tr	Tr
Taro, cooked, sliced	1 cup	190	46	7	39	Tr	Tr
Taro Chips	1 oz	140	19	2	17	Tr	7
Taro Leaf, steamed	½ cup	15	3	2	1	2	Tr
Tarragon	...	...	.	.	.	.	.
Dried, leaves	1 tsp	0	Tr	0	Tr	Tr	Tr
Dried, ground	1 tsp	5	Tr	Tr	Tr	Tr	Tr
T-bone Steak – see Beef	...	...	.	.	.	.	.
Thyme	...	...	.	.	.	.	.
Dried, leaves	1 tsp	0	Tr	Tr	Tr	Tr	Tr
Dried, ground	1 tsp	0	Tr	Tr	Tr	Tr	Tr
Fresh	1 tsp	0	Tr	Tr	Tr	Tr	Tr
Toaster Pastry (Pop Tart)	...	...	.	.	.	.	.
Apple, frosted	1 pastry	220	39	Tr	39	2	6
Apple, unfrosted	1 pastry	210	37	Tr	37	2	6
Blueberry, frosted	1 pastry	220	39	Tr	39	2	6
Blueberry, unfrosted	1 pastry	210	37	Tr	37	2	6
Brown sugar cinnamon	1 pastry	210	34	Tr	34	3	7
Cherry, frosted	1 pastry	220	39	Tr	39	2	6
Cherry, unfrosted	1 pastry	210	37	Tr	37	2	6
Strawberry, frosted	1 pastry	220	39	Tr	39	2	6
Strawberry, unfrosted	1 pastry	210	37	Tr	37	2	6
Tofu, raw	½ cup	90	2	Tr	2	10	6
Tomatillos, raw	...	...	.	.	.	.	.
Whole, medium size	2	20	4	1	3	Tr	Tr
Chopped or diced	½ cup	20	4	1	3	Tr	Tr
Tomato	...	...	.	.	.	.	.
Fresh, raw, avg size 2 ½" dia	1 whole	20	5	2	3	1	Tr

	SERVING SIZE	CALORIES	TOTAL CARBS (g)	FIBER (g)	NET CARBS (g)	PROTEIN (g)	FAT (g)
Fresh, raw, cherry tomato	1 cup	25	6	2	4	1	Tr
Fresh, slices, ¼" thick	1 slice	0	Tr	Tr	Tr	Tr	Tr
Fresh, chopped or sliced	1 cup	30	7	2	5	2	Tr
Fresh, cooked	1 cup	45	10	2	8	2	Tr
Fresh, stewed	1 cup	80	13	2	11	2	3
Canned, packed in juice	1 cup	40	10	2	8	2	Tr
Canned, stewed	1 cup	70	16	3	13	2	Tr
Sun Dried	...	...	.	.	.	.	.
Plain	1 piece	5	1	Tr	1	Tr	Tr
Packed in oil, drained	1 piece	5	Tr	Tr	Tr	Tr	Tr
Tomato Paste	1 Tbsp	15	3	Tr	3	Tr	Tr
Tomato Puree	1 cup	100	23	5	18	4	Tr
Tomato Sauce, canned	1 cup	60	13	4	9	3	Tr
Topping, for dessert	...	...	.	.	.	.	.
Butterscotch, regular	2 Tbsp	100	27	Tr	27	Tr	Tr
Caramel	2 Tbsp	100	27	Tr	27	Tr	Tr
Cream, Whipped Topping	...	...	.	.	.	.	.
Light cream	1 cup	350	4	0	4	3	37
Light cream	2 Tbsp	45	Tr	0	Tr	Tr	5
Heavy cream	1 cup	410	3	0	3	3	44
Heavy cream	2 Tbsp	50	Tr	0	Tr	Tr	6
Pressurized in can	1 Tbsp	10	Tr	0	Tr	Tr	Tr
Marshmallow cream	1 oz	90	22	0	22	Tr	Tr
Pineapple	2 Tbsp	110	28	Tr	28	Tr	Tr
Strawberry Topping	2 Tbsp	110	28	Tr	28	Tr	Tr

	SERVING SIZE	CALORIES	TOTAL CARBS (g)	FIBER (g)	NET CARBS (g)	PROTEIN (g)	FAT (g)
Tortellini	...	...	.	.	.	.	.
Cheese filling	¾ cup	250	38	2	36	11	6
Tortilla, 6" dia, ready to cook	...	...	.	.	.	.	.
Corn	1	50	11	2	9	1	Tr
Flour	1	90	15	Tr	15	3	2
Tortilla Chips	...	...	.	.	.	.	.
Regular, yellow corn	1 oz	140	19	1	18	2	6
Regular, white corn	1 oz	140	19	2	17	2	7
Lowfat, baked	1 oz	120	23	2	21	3	2
Nacho flavor, regular	1 oz	150	18	1	17	2	7
Nacho flavor, reduced fat, baked	1 oz	125	20	1	19	2	4
(also see Corn Chips)	...	...	.	.	.	.	.
Tostada – see individual restaurant listings	...	...	.	.	.	.	.
Tuna – see Fish	...	...	.	.	.	.	.
Tuna Dishes – see Frozen Dinner	...	...	.	.	.	.	.
Tuna Salad	½ cup	190	10	0	10	16	10
TURKEY	...	...	.	.	.	.	.
Roast Turkey	...	...	.	.	.	.	.
light & dark meat	3 oz	150	0	0	0	25	4
light meat only	3 oz	130	0	0	0	25	3
dark meat only	3 oz	160	0	0	0	24	6
Giblets, simmered, chopped	1 cup	290	1	0	1	30	17
Ground Turkey, 4 oz patty, cooked	1	190	0	0	0	22	11
Neck, simmered	3 oz	150	0	0	0	23	6

	SERVING SIZE	CALORIES	TOTAL CARBS (g)	FIBER (g)	NET CARBS (g)	PROTEIN (g)	FAT (g)
(Other Turkey Products, see:	...	...	.	.	.	.	.
Bologna, Hot Dog, Salami,	...	...	.	.	.	.	.
Sausage & specific entrées)	...	...	.	.	.	.	.
Turmeric, ground	1 tsp	10	1	Tr	1	Tr	Tr
Turnip, cooked	...	...	.	.	.	.	.
Cubes	½ cup	15	4	2	2	Tr	Tr
Mashed	½ cup	25	6	2	4	Tr	Tr
Turnip Greens, cooked, chopped	1 cup	30	6	5	1	1	Tr
Vanilla Extract	...	...	.	.	.	.	.
Real or imitation	1 tsp	10	Tr	0	Tr	0	0
Alcohol-free	1 tsp	0	Tr	0	Tr	0	0
Veal	...	...	.	.	.	.	.
Chop, loin, braised	...	...	.	.	.	.	.
lean & fat	3 oz	240	0	0	0	26	15
lean only	3 oz	190	0	0	0	29	8
Leg (top round), braised, lean & fat	3 oz	180	0	0	0	31	5
Liver, braised	3 oz	160	0	0	0	24	5
Rib, roasted	...	...	.	.	.	.	.
lean & fat	3 oz	190	0	0	0	20	12
lean only	3 oz	150	0	0	0	22	6
Shank, braised	...	...	.	.	.	.	.
lean & fat	3 oz	160	0	0	0	27	5
lean only	3 oz	150	0	0	0	27	4
Shoulder, braised	...	...	.	.	.	.	.
lean & fat	3 oz	190	0	0	0	27	9
lean only	3 oz	170	0	0	0	29	5
Vegetable Burger	1 patty	120	10	3	7	11	4

	SERVING SIZE	CALORIES	TOTAL CARBS (g)	FIBER (g)	NET CARBS (g)	PROTEIN (g)	FAT (g)
Vegetables, mixed	...	...	.	.	.	.	.
(See specific listings for individual vegetables)	...	...	.	.	.	.	.
Mixed, canned, drained, heated	1 cup	80	15	5	10	4	Tr
Frozen, cooked	1 cup	120	24	8	16	5	Tr
Vinegar	...	...	.	.	.	.	.
Balsamic	1 Tbsp	15	3	Tr	3	Tr	0
Distilled	1 Tbsp	0	Tr	0	Tr	0	0
Cider vinegar	1 Tbsp	0	Tr	0	Tr	0	0
Red wine	1 Tbsp	0	Tr	0	Tr	Tr	0
Waffle	...	...	.	.	.	.	.
Frozen, plain, 4" dia	1	100	16	Tr	16	2	3
Frozen, buttermilk, 4" dia	1	100	16	Tr	16	3	3
Walnut – see Nuts	...	...	.	.	.	.	.
Water Chestnut, canned, slices	½ cup	35	9	2	7	Tr	Tr
Watercress, raw, chopped	½ cup	0	Tr	Tr	Tr	Tr	Tr
Raw, sprigs	10	0	Tr	Tr	Tr	Tr	Tr
Watermelon	...	...	.	.	.	.	.
Fresh, diced or balls	1 cup	45	12	Tr	12	Tr	Tr
Fresh, wedge, 1" thick, 1⁄16 of melon 15" long × 7 ½" dia	1 wedge	90	22	1	21	2	Tr
Wheat Bran	¼ cup	30	9	6	3	2	Tr
Wheat Germ, toasted, plain	1 Tbsp	25	4	1	3	2	Tr
Whipped Cream – see Cream	...	...	.	.	.	.	.

	SERVING SIZE	CALORIES	TOTAL CARBS (g)	FIBER (g)	NET CARBS (g)	PROTEIN (g)	FAT (g)
Wiener – see Hot Dog	...	...	.	.	.	.	.
Yam – see Sweet Potato	...	...	.	.	.	.	.
Yeast	...	...	.	.	.	.	.
Compressed	1 cake	20	3	1	2	1	Tr
Dry, active, regular size pkg	1	20	3	2	1	3	Tr
Dry, active	1 tsp	10	2	Tr	2	2	Tr
Yeast Extract Spread	1 tsp	10	Tr	Tr	Tr	Tr	0
Yogurt	...	...	.	.	.	.	.
Vanilla, lowfat	½ cup	100	17	0	17	6	2
Yogurt, plain,	...	...	.	.	.	.	.
made w/ whole milk	½ cup	80	6	0	6	4	4
made w/ lowfat milk	½ cup	80	9	0	9	6	2
made w/ skim milk	½ cup	70	9	0	9	7	Tr
Yogurt, fruit, lowfat	½ cup	120	23	0	23	5	1
Yogurt, fruit, nonfat	½ cup	120	23	0	23	5	Tr
Yogurt, fruit, w/low calorie sweetener	½ cup	130	23	0	23	6	2
Yogurt, Frozen	...	...	.	.	.	.	.
Regular	½ cup	110	19	0	19	3	3
Regular, Chocolate	½ cup	110	19	1	18	3	3
Vanilla, soft serve	½ cup	120	17	0	17	3	4
Chocolate, soft serve	½ cup	120	18	2	16	3	4
Zucchini	...	...	.	.	.	.	.
Fresh, med size	1	30	7	2	5	2	Tr

FAST FOOD RESTAURANTS

	SERVING SIZE	CALORIES	TOTAL CARBS (g)	FIBER (g)	NET CARBS (g)	PROTEIN (g)	FAT (g)
A&W	...	...	.	.	.	.	.
A&W diet root beer float	16 oz	170	30	0	30	2	5
A&W diet root beer, large	22 fl oz	0	0	0	0	0	0
A&W diet root beer, medium	14 fl oz	0	0	0	0	0	0
A&W diet root beer, small	11 fl oz	0	0	0	0	0	0
A&W regular root beer, large	22 fl oz	460	121	0	121	0	0
A&W regular root beer, medium	14 fl oz	290	76	0	76	0	0
A&W regular root beer, small	11 fl oz	220	57	0	57	0	0
A&W root beer float	16 oz	330	70	0	70	2	5
A&W root beer freeze	16 oz	430	79	0	79	9	9
BBQ dipping sauce	1 oz	40	10	0	10	0	0
Breaded onion rings, large	1	480	62	3	59	7	27
Breaded onion rings, regular	1	350	45	2	43	5	16
Burger patty, extra	1	170	2	0	2	15	12
Caramel sundae	1	340	57	0	57	8	9
Cheese curds	1	570	27	2	25	27	40
Cheese fries	1	390	50	4	46	4	18
Cheeseburger	1	420	37	4	33	23	21
Chicken strips	3 pc	500	32	2	30	28	29
Chili cheese fries	1	410	52	5	47	8	17
Chocolate milkshake	16 oz	700	100	2	98	11	29

	SERVING SIZE	CALORIES	TOTAL CARBS (g)	FIBER (g)	NET CARBS (g)	PROTEIN (g)	FAT (g)
A&W (cont.)	...	...	.	.	.	.	.
Chocolate sundae	1	320	53	0	53	8	8
Coney (chili) cheese dog	1	380	28	2	26	14	23
Coney (chili) dog	1	340	26	2	24	14	20
Corn dog nuggets, regular	8 pc	280	32	2	30	9	13
Corn dog nuggets, small	5 pc	180	20	1	19	5	8
Crispy chicken sandwich	1	550	52	5	47	30	25
French fries, large	1	430	61	6	55	5	17
French fries, regular	1	310	45	4	41	3	12
French fries, small	1	200	28	3	25	2	8
Grilled chicken sandwich	1	400	31	4	27	35	15
Hamburger	1	380	33	3	30	21	19
Honey mustard dipping sauce	1 oz	100	12	0	12	0	6
Hot dog, plain	1	310	23	1	22	11	19
Hot fudge sundae	1	350	54	1	53	8	11
M&M's Polar Swirl	12 oz	710	107	2	105	15	25
Oreo Polar Swirl	12 oz	690	107	3	104	14	24
Original bacon cheeseburger	1	530	39	4	35	26	30
Original Bacon double cheeseburger	1	760	45	4	41	44	45
Original double cheeseburger	1	680	44	4	40	40	38
Papa Burger	1	690	44	4	40	40	39
Papa Single Burger	1	470	38	4	34	23	25
Ranch dipping sauce	1 oz	160	2	0	2	0	17
Reese's Polar Swirl	12 oz	740	97	3	94	18	31

	SERVING SIZE	CALORIES	TOTAL CARBS (g)	FIBER (g)	NET CARBS (g)	PROTEIN (g)	FAT (g)
A&W (cont.)	. . .	. . .	.	.	.	.	.
Strawberry milkshake	16 oz	670	90	0	90	11	29
Strawberry sundae	1	300	47	0	47	12	8
Vanilla cone	16 oz	260	41	0	41	7	7
Vanilla milkshake	16 oz	720	97	0	97	12	31
Arby's	. . .	. . .	.	.	.	.	.
All American Roastburger	1	420	46	2	44	19	18
Apple turnover, no icing	1	250	35	2	33	4	14
Arby's Melt	1	300	36	2	34	16	12
Bacon & Bleu Roastburger	1	470	44	2	42	22	23
bacon, add on	1	80	1	0	1	5	6
Balsamic vinaigrette dressing	1 svg	130	5	0	5	0	12
BBQ sauce	1 svg	45	11	0	11	0	0
Beef 'n cheddar sandwich, large	1	660	46	3	43	43	36
Beef 'n cheddar sandwich, medium	1	540	44	2	42	33	27
Beef 'n cheddar sandwich, regular	1	440	43	2	41	22	20
Buffalo sauce	1 svg	10	2	0	2	0	1
Buttermilk ranch dressing	1 svg	230	2	0	2	0	24
Cheddar cheese sauce for curly fries	1 svg	50	4	0	4	1	4
Cherry turnover, no icing	1	250	35	2	33	4	14
Chicken cordon bleu, crispy	1	570	47	2	45	36	25
Chicken cordon bleu, roast	1	460	37	2	35	33	18

	SERVING SIZE	CALORIES	TOTAL CARBS (g)	FIBER (g)	NET CARBS (g)	PROTEIN (g)	FAT (g)
Arby's (cont.)	...	...	.	.	.	.	.
Chicken fillet sandwich, crispy	1	480	47	2	45	25	23
Chicken fillet sandwich, roast	1	380	37	2	35	23	16
Chicken, bacon & swiss sandwich, crispy	1	540	50	2	48	31	23
Chicken, bacon & swiss sandwich, roast	1	440	40	2	38	30	16
Chocolate swirl shake	1	650	110	Tr	110	16	17
Chopped farmhouse chicken salad, crispy	1	390	26	4	22	25	19
Chopped farmhouse chicken salad, grilled	1	250	10	3	7	22	12
Chopped Italian salad	1	430	11	3	8	23	31
Chopped turkey club salad	1	250	10	3	7	23	12
Classic Italian toasted sub	1	600	61	3	58	25	27
Corned beef reuben sandwich	1	610	55	3	52	34	33
Curly fries, large	1	600	70	7	63	8	36
Curly fries, medium	1	500	58	6	52	7	29
Curly fries, small	1	360	42	4	38	5	21
Dijon honey mustard dressing	1 svg	150	8	0	8	1	17
French dip & swiss toasted sub w/ au jus	1	510	63	3	60	29	16
Ham & Swiss Melt	1	280	35	1	34	18	6

	SERVING SIZE	CALORIES	TOTAL CARBS (g)	FIBER (g)	NET CARBS (g)	PROTEIN (g)	FAT (g)
A&W (cont.)	...	...	.	.	.	.	.
Icing for turnovers	1 svg	130	29	0	29	0	2
Jalapeno bites, large	8 pc	490	47	3	44	9	34
Jalapeno bites, regular	5 pc	310	29	2	27	5	21
Jamocha swirl shake	1	640	107	Tr	107	16	17
Loaded potato bites, large	8 pc	570	43	4	39	18	35
Loaded potato bites, regular	5 pc	350	27	2	25	11	22
Mozzarella sticks, large	6 pc	640	57	3	54	27	42
Mozzarella sticks, regular	4 pc	430	38	2	36	18	28
Pecan chicken salad sandwich	1	870	92	6	86	25	47
Philly beef toasted sub	1	590	59	3	48	29	26
Popcorn chicken, large	1	410	34	3	31	27	18
Popcorn chicken, regular	1	330	27	2	25	22	15
Potato cakes, large	4	490	52	5	47	3	37
Potato cakes, medium	3	370	39	3	36	3	28
Potato cakes, small	2	250	26	2	24	2	18
Roast beef & swiss sandwich	1	760	73	6	67	35	40
Roast beef sandwich, large	1	550	41	3	38	42	28
Roast beef sandwich, medium	1	415	34	2	32	31	21
Roast beef sandwich, regular	1	320	34	2	32	21	14

	SERVING SIZE	CALORIES	TOTAL CARBS (g)	FIBER (g)	NET CARBS (g)	PROTEIN (g)	FAT (g)
Arby's (cont.)	...	...	.	.	.	.	.
Roast chicken club	1	500	46	2	44	30	17
Roast ham & swiss sandwich	1	690	75	5	70	33	31
Roast turkey & swiss sandwich	1	710	74	5	69	41	30
Roast turkey, ranch & bacon sandwich	1	820	74	5	69	46	38
Super Roast Beef	1	400	41	2	39	21	19
Turkey bacon club toasted sub	1	580	60	3	57	35	21
Ultimate BLT sandwich	1	780	75	6	69	23	45
Vanilla shake	1	550	83	0	83	16	17
Au Bon Pain	...	...	.	.	.	.	.
Almond croissant	1	600	55	4	51	13	38
Apple croissant	1	280	44	3	41	5	11
Apple croissants tart	1 oz	80	12	1	11	1	4
Apple streudel	1	440	50	1	49	5	24
Arizona chicken sandwich	1	690	60	4	56	47	28
Asiago cheese bagel	1	340	56	2	54	15	6
Bacon & bagel sandwich	1	340	58	2	56	16	6
Bacon & egg melt sandwich, on ciabatta	1	510	41	2	39	26	26
Baja turkey sandwich	1	700	71	5	66	46	27
Baked potato	1 oz	25	5	1	4	1	0
Baked stuffed potato soup	12 oz	350	29	2	27	9	20
Balsamic vinaigrette dressing	2 oz	120	8	0	8	0	9

	SERVING SIZE	CALORIES	TOTAL CARBS (g)	FIBER (g)	NET CARBS (g)	PROTEIN (g)	FAT (g)
Au Bon Pain (cont.)	...	...	.	.	.	.	.
Banana nut pound cake	1	480	56	1	55	7	26
BBQ beef salad	1 oz	35	4	0	4	2	1
BBQ brisket harvest rice bowl	1	790	118	10	108	37	19
BBQ brisket harvest rice bowl w/ brown rice	1	740	103	12	91	37	21
BBQ brisket sandwich	1	660	81	5	76	36	21
BBQ brisket wrap	1	690	82	8	74	32	28
BBQ chicken & beef stew	12 oz	300	35	3	32	19	10
BBQ chicken harvest rice bowl	1	690	120	12	108	31	11
BBQ chicken harvest rice bowl w/ brown rice	1	650	105	13	92	31	12
BBQ chicken sandwich	1	560	83	6	77	29	13
BBQ chicken wrap	1	640	83	9	74	29	24
Beef & vegetable stew	12 oz	310	25	3	22	18	16
Beef stroganoff penne	1 oz	40	4	0	4	2	2
Black bean soup	12 oz	260	46	26	20	15	1
Blondie	1	460	59	2	57	5	33
Blue cheese dressing	2 oz	310	2	0	2	2	33
Blueberry muffin	1	490	74	2	72	9	17
Broccoli cheddar soup	12 oz	300	20	2	18	11	21
Brown rice	1 oz	30	6	0	6	1	0
Brown rice Waldorf salad	1 oz	45	5	0	5	0	3

	SERVING SIZE	CALORIES	TOTAL CARBS (g)	FIBER (g)	NET CARBS (g)	PROTEIN (g)	FAT (g)
Au Bon Pain (cont.)	...	...	.	.	.	.	.
Caesar dressing	2 oz	270	4	0	4	1	28
Caprese sandwich	1	680	65	4	61	30	32
Carrot ginger soup	12 oz	140	22	3	19	1	5
Carrot walnut muffin	1	560	72	4	68	9	27
Chef's salad	1	250	7	3	4	24	15
Cherry danish	1	420	54	1	53	7	20
Cherry streudel	1	460	50	1	49	5	26
Chicken & dumpling soup	12 oz	210	28	2	26	11	7
Chicken & vegetable stew	12 oz	290	26	3	23	11	17
Chicken broccoli alfredo penne	1 oz	60	3	0	3	2	4
Chicken broccoli alfredo penne	12 oz	680	38	2	36	28	43
Chicken caesar asiago wrap	1	610	61	5	56	34	28
Chicken florentine soup	12 oz	250	25	1	24	8	13
Chicken gumbo	12 oz	180	21	2	19	6	8
Chicken marsala penne	1 oz	35	4	0	4	2	1
Chicken noodle soup	12 oz	130	19	2	17	8	3
Chicken penne pesto	1 oz	60	4	0	4	3	3
Chicken pesto sandwich	1	660	66	4	62	43	24
Chicken provençal	1 oz	25	4	0	4	2	0
Chickpea & tomato cucumber salad	1	230	23	7	16	11	12
Chocolate cheesecake brownie	1	460	74	1	73	5	19

	SERVING SIZE	CALORIES	TOTAL CARBS (g)	FIBER (g)	NET CARBS (g)	PROTEIN (g)	FAT (g)
Au Bon Pain (cont.)	...	...	.	.	.	.	.
Chocolate cherry tulip	1	410	54	2	52	5	21
Chocolate chip brownie	1	510	74	1	73	6	19
Chocolate chip cookie	1	280	40	2	38	3	13
Chocolate chip muffin	1	580	83	3	80	9	23
Chocolate croissant	1	440	58	3	55	7	22
Chocolate dipped cranberry almond macaroon	1	300	36	4	32	4	15
Chocolate dipped shortbread	1	380	42	1	41	4	22
Chocolate orange pecan scone	1	580	74	3	71	10	28
Cinnamon crisp bagel	1	410	77	4	73	11	7
Cinnamon raisin bagel	1	320	68	3	65	11	1
Cinnamon scone	1	530	60	2	58	9	27
Cinnamon walnut quinoa	1 oz	45	4	1	3	2	3
Clam chowder	12 oz	320	27	1	26	9	18
Confetti cookie w/ *M&M's*	1	280	39	0	39	3	13
Corn & green chili bisque	12 oz	260	27	3	24	6	15
Corn chowder	12 oz	350	40	3	37	9	18
Corn muffin	1	490	75	3	72	10	17
Cranberry walnut muffin	1	540	66	4	62	10	25
Cream of chicken & wild rice soup	12 oz	240	22	1	21	6	14
Creamed spinach	1 oz	30	2	1	1	1	2

	SERVING SIZE	CALORIES	TOTAL CARBS (g)	FIBER (g)	NET CARBS (g)	PROTEIN (g)	FAT (g)
Au Bon Pain (cont.)	...	...	.	.	.	.	.
Crème de fleur	1	500	57	2	55	11	25
Crumb cake	1	750	97	1	96	8	40
Curried rice & lentil soup	12 oz	170	30	8	22	8	2
Demi chicken sandwich w/ cheddar, on baguette	1	440	50	3	47	27	15
Demi chicken sandwich, on baguette	1	370	49	3	46	22	9
Demi ham sandwich w/ swiss, on baguette	1	400	56	3	53	23	10
Demi ham sandwich, on baguette	1	330	56	3	53	17	5
Demi roast beef sandwich w/ brie, on baguette	1	460	49	3	46	24	18
Demi roast beef sandwich, on baguette	1	360	49	3	46	19	8
Demi tuna sandwich w/ cheddar, on baguette	1	400	50	3	47	22	14
Demi tuna sandwich, on baguette	1	320	49	3	46	17	7
Demi turkey sandwich w/ swiss, on baguette	1	400	49	2	47	24	12
Demi turkey sandwich, on baguette	1	320	49	2	47	18	6

	SERVING SIZE	CALORIES	TOTAL CARBS (g)	FIBER (g)	NET CARBS (g)	PROTEIN (g)	FAT (g)
Au Bon Pain (cont.)	. . .	. . .	.	.	.	.	.
Double chocolate chunk muffin	1	620	86	4	82	11	25
Egg & bacon bagel sandwich	1	420	60	3	57	25	8
Egg & broccoli baked sandwich	1	350	42	3	39	23	10
Egg & cheese bagel sandwich	1	450	61	3	58	26	10
Egg & cucumber salad	1 oz	40	1	0	1	2	3
Egg bagel sandwich	1	360	60	3	57	21	4
Egg, bacon & cheese bagel sandwich	1	510	61	3	58	31	15
Eggplant & mozzarella sandwich	1	670	73	6	67	27	30
Eggplant parmesan	1 oz	50	4	1	3	2	3
English toffee cake	1	250	27	1	26	2	14
Everything bagel	1	340	61	3	58	13	5
Fat free raspberry vinaigrette	2 oz	50	12	0	12	0	0
Fire roasted exotic grains & vegetables	1 oz	40	7	1	6	1	1
French Moroccan tomato lentil soup	12 oz	190	32	10	22	10	2
French onion soup	12 oz	130	19	2	17	3	5
French pecan toast	1 oz	70	8	0	8	2	4
Garden salad	1	70	12	3	9	3	2
Garden vegetable soup	12 oz	80	13	3	10	3	2
Gazpacho	12 oz	90	11	3	8	2	5

	SERVING SIZE	CALORIES	TOTAL CARBS (g)	FIBER (g)	NET CARBS (g)	PROTEIN (g)	FAT (g)
Au Bon Pain (cont.)	. . .	. . .	.	.	.	.	.
Grilled chicken Caesar asiago salad	1	300	18	3	15	28	13
Ham & cheese croissant	1	400	38	2	36	15	20
Ham & swiss half sandwich, on farmhouse roll	1	320	34	2	32	21	13
Ham & swiss sandwich, on country white bread	1	530	60	2	58	39	17
Hazelnut Mocha brownie	1	490	74	3	71	6	22
Hazelnut vinaigrette dressing	2 oz	270	11	0	11	1	25
Hearty cabbage soup	12 oz	110	14	3	11	5	5
Honey 9 grain bagel	1	350	69	6	63	12	4
Honey pecan cream cheese	2 oz	200	10	0	10	2	16
Iced cinnamon roll	1	410	60	2	58	8	15
Italian sausage, peppers & onions	1 oz	25	1	0	1	2	1
Italian wedding soup	12 oz	170	19	3	16	8	7
Jalapeno double cheddar bagel	1	340	53	2	51	17	10
Jalapeno mayonnaise	1 oz	50	1	0	1	2	5
Jamaican black bean soup	12 oz	250	43	23	20	16	1
Jambalaya	1 oz	25	2	0	2	1	1
Lemon danish	1	440	57	1	56	7	20
Lemon drop tulip	1	410	55	1	54	5	19

	SERVING SIZE	CALORIES	TOTAL CARBS (g)	FIBER (g)	NET CARBS (g)	PROTEIN (g)	FAT (g)
Au Bon Pain (cont.)	. . .	. . .	.	.	.	.	.
Lemon pound cake	1	520	67	1	66	6	25
Light ranch dressing	2 oz	120	3	0	3	2	11
Lite cream cheese spread	2 oz	120	5	0	5	4	9
Lite honey mustard dressing	2 oz	170	20	0	20	1	9
Lite olive oil vinaigrette	2 oz	110	6	0	6	0	10
Low-fat triple berry muffin	1	300	65	2	63	4	3
Macaroni & cheese	1 oz	40	3	0	3	2	3
Macaroni & cheese	12 oz	500	36	2	34	20	29
Mandarin sesame chicken salad	1	310	29	3	26	20	17
Marble pound cake	1	490	59	1	58	6	26
Mayan chicken harvest rice bowl	1	560	87	5	82	27	12
Mayan chicken harvest rice bowl w/ brown rice	1	510	72	7	65	27	13
Mayan chicken hot wrap	1	580	93	6	87	24	13
Mayonnaise	1 oz	70	2	0	2	0	7
Meat lasagna	1 oz	45	4	0	4	2	2
Meat lasagna	10.7 oz	470	41	5	36	22	24
Meatballs & marinara sauce	1 oz	50	2	1	1	2	4
Meatloaf w/ wine sauce	1 oz	50	2	0	2	2	3
Mediterranean chicken salad	1	290	12	3	9	23	16
Mediterranean spread	1 oz	120	2	1	1	2	11
Mediterranean wrap	1	610	73	8	65	18	29

	SERVING SIZE	CALORIES	TOTAL CARBS (g)	FIBER (g)	NET CARBS (g)	PROTEIN (g)	FAT (g)
Au Bon Pain (cont.)	...	...	.	.	.	.	.
Mediterranean pepper soup	12 oz	170	26	8	18	7	5
Mini chocolate chip cookie	1	70	10	0	10	1	3
Mini oatmeal raisin cookie	1	60	10	1	9	1	3
Mint chocolate pound cake	1	530	64	3	61	7	29
Mozzarella chicken sandwich	1	680	67	4	63	48	24
Mustard	1 tsp	0	0	0	0	0	0
Oatmeal raisin cookie	1	230	36	2	34	3	8
Oatmeal, medium	12 oz	210	38	5	33	8	4
Old fashioned tomato soup	12 oz	200	27	3	24	6	7
Onion dill bagel	1	280	57	3	54	11	1
Orange scone	1	470	57	1	56	10	23
Orzo toscano salad	1 oz	35	6	1	5	1	1
Palmier	1	440	53	1	52	1	23
Pasta e fagioli soup	12 oz	260	35	9	26	12	8
Pecan roll	1	810	99	3	96	12	41
Penne marinara	1 oz	30	55	5	50	1	1
Pineapple blueberry cobbler	1 oz	45	8	1	7	1	2
Plain bagel	1	280	56	2	54	11	1
Plain croissant	1	310	31	1	30	7	17
Polenta marinara	1 oz	25	3	0	3	1	1
Pomegranate vinaigrette dressing	2 oz	250	12	0	12	0	22
Poppy bagel	1	320	58	4	54	12	4
Portobello & goat cheese sandwich	1	550	62	6	56	19	25

	SERVING SIZE	CALORIES	TOTAL CARBS (g)	FIBER (g)	NET CARBS (g)	PROTEIN (g)	FAT (g)
Au Bon Pain (cont.)	...	...	.	.	.	.	.
Portobello, egg & cheddar sandwich	1	500	42	3	39	22	26
Portuguese kale soup	12 oz	130	15	4	11	5	5
Potato bacon salad	1 oz	40	5	1	4	1	2
Potato cheese soup	12 oz	260	24	2	22	7	14
Potato leek soup	12 oz	300	28	2	26	5	19
Prosciutto & egg sandwich, on asiago bagel	1	520	60	1	59	34	16
Prosciutto mozzarella sandwich	1	810	71	4	67	41	41
Quinoa	1 oz	25	4	1	3	1	0
Raisin bran muffin	1	480	85	10	75	12	11
Raspberry cheese croissant	1	370	46	2	44	8	17
Red beans, italian sausage & rice soup	12 oz	270	40	17	23	14	6
Roast beef & brie half sandwich, on farmhouse roll	1	350	34	2	32	20	14
Roast beef & brie sandwich, on country white bread	1	600	59	3	56	39	21
Roast beef caesar sandwich	1	680	68	3	65	40	27
Roasted apple cranberry orzo	1 oz	45	9	1	8	1	1
Roasted carrots	1 oz	15	3	1	2	0	0
Roasted greens beans w/ almonds	1 oz	20	2	1	1	1	1
Roasted potatoes	1 oz	35	6	1	5	1	2

	SERVING SIZE	CALORIES	TOTAL CARBS (g)	FIBER (g)	NET CARBS (g)	PROTEIN (g)	FAT (g)
Au Bon Pain (cont.)	. . .	. . .	.	.	.	.	.
Roasted zucchini & summer squash	1 oz	5	1	0	1	0	0
Rocky road brownie	1	490	74	2	72	6	22
Sausage w/ peppers & onions	1 oz	50	1	0	1	2	5
Sausage, egg & cheddar sandwich, on asiago bagel	1	810	58	1	57	38	47
Scrambled eggs	1 oz	35	1	0	1	3	3
Sesame brown rice & orange salad	1 oz	45	6	0	6	1	3
Sesame ginger dressing	2 oz	230	12	0	12	1	20
Sesame seed bagel	1	330	59	3	56	12	5
Shortbread cookie	1	340	37	1	36	4	20
Side garden salad	1	50	8	2	6	2	1
Smoked salmon & wasabi sandwich, on onion dill bagel	1	430	64	1	63	23	11
Southern black-eyed pea soup	12 oz	170	29	9	20	11	2
Southwest corn casserole	1 oz	60	4	0	4	3	4
Southwest fusilli pasta salad	1 oz	45	4	0	4	1	3
Southwest jalapeno muffin	1	560	64	2	62	8	30
Southwest panzanella salad	1 oz	50	7	0	7	1	3
Southwest tortilla soup	12 oz	190	23	4	19	4	10
Southwest tuna wrap	1	750	66	7	59	39	40
Southwest vegetable soup	12 oz	170	37	8	29	8	5

	SERVING SIZE	CALORIES	TOTAL CARBS (g)	FIBER (g)	NET CARBS (g)	PROTEIN (g)	FAT (g)
Au Bon Pain (cont.)	...	...	.	.	.	.	.
Spicy tuna sandwich	1	470	60	11	49	29	16
Spinach & cheese croissant	1	290	28	2	26	10	16
Split pea w/ ham soup	12 oz	250	41	15	26	18	2
Steakhouse sandwich, on ciabatta	1	720	76	4	72	44	30
Stuffed peppers w/ lentils	1 oz	20	3	1	2	1	0
Sundried tomato cream cheese	2 oz	140	5	1	4	4	11
Sun-dried tomato spread	0.5 oz	45	1	0	1	0	4
Sweet cheese croissant	1	400	49	1	48	9	19
Sweet cheese Danish	1	470	54	1	53	9	24
Thai coconut curry soup	12 oz	160	21	2	19	4	7
Thai peanut chicken salad	1	240	19	4	15	22	8
Thai peanut chicken wrap	1	530	79	6	73	30	15
Thai peanut dressing	2 oz	160	20	0	20	2	8
Tomato basil bisque	12 oz	210	27	4	23	7	9
Tomato cheddar soup	12 oz	240	17	2	15	8	16
Tomato cucumber salad	1 oz	10	2	0	2	0	0
Tomato florentine soup	12 oz	130	18	2	16	6	3
Tomato rice soup	12 oz	120	24	2	22	4	1

	SERVING SIZE	CALORIES	TOTAL CARBS (g)	FIBER (g)	NET CARBS (g)	PROTEIN (g)	FAT (g)
Au Bon Pain (cont.)	...	...	.	.	.	.	.
Tomato, green bean & almond salad	1 oz	20	2	0	2	0	2
Tsaziki	1 oz	15	2	0	2	1	0
Tuna & cheddar half sandwich, on farmhouse roll	1	360	35	2	33	19	16
Tuna & cheddar sandwich, on country white bread	1	610	63	3	60	37	25
Tuna garden salad	1	240	15	4	11	20	12
Tuna melt	1	690	71	5	66	42	30
Tuna salad	1 oz	40	1	0	1	4	3
Turkey & strawberry salad	1	110	10	4	6	11	4
Turkey & swiss half sandwich, on farmhouse roll	1	320	34	2	32	22	11
Turkey & swiss sandwich, on country white bread	1	530	60	2	58	42	14
Turkey club sandwich	1	700	59	2	57	45	31
Turkey cobb salad	1	330	14	4	10	27	19
Turkey melt	1	810	79	3	76	47	32
Tuscan vegetable soup	12 oz	170	23	3	20	7	5
Vegetable beef barley soup	12 oz	140	21	4	17	9	3
Vegetable cream cheese	2 oz	170	3	0	3	3	16
Vegetarian chili	12 oz	220	39	20	19	12	2
Vegetarian lasagna	1 oz	20	4	1	3	1	0
Vegetarian lentil soup	12 oz	170	31	11	20	9	2

	SERVING SIZE	CALORIES	TOTAL CARBS (g)	FIBER (g)	NET CARBS (g)	PROTEIN (g)	FAT (g)
Au Bon Pain (cont.)	...	...	.	.	.	.	.
Vegetarian minestrone soup	12 oz	120	20	4	16	5	2
Watermelon & feta salad	1 oz	15	3	0	3	0	1
White chocolate chunk macadamia nut cookie	1	300	36	1	35	3	16
White chocolate toffee bagel braid	1	350	63	2	61	11	6
White rice	1 oz	35	8	0	8	1	0
Wild mushroom bisque	12 oz	190	22	2	20	5	9
Baskin Robbins	*(all ice creams one small scoop, unless noted)*	...	.	.	.	.	.
Aloha Brownie, light churned	1	150	26	1	25	3	5
Butter Almond Crunch, reduced fat, no sugar added	1	140	19	3	16	4	7
Cabana Berry Banana, reduced fat, no sugar added	1	90	17	2	15	3	4
Cake Cone	1	25	5	0	5	0	0
Cappuccino Chip, light churned	1	140	20	1	19	3	5
Caramel Turtle Truffle, reduced fat, no sugar added	1	120	24	2	22	3	5
Cherries Jubilee	1	150	19	1	18	3	8

	SERVING SIZE	CALORIES	TOTAL CARBS (g)	FIBER (g)	NET CARBS (g)	PROTEIN (g)	FAT (g)
Baskin Robbins (cont.)	...	...	.	.	.	.	.
Chocolate Chip Cookie Dough	1	190	23	0	23	3	9
Chocolate chip ice cream	1	170	17	0	17	3	10
Chocolate Fudge	1	160	21	0	21	3	10
Chocolate ice cream	1	160	21	0	21	3	9
Chocolate Overload, reduced fat, no sugar added	1	120	23	3	20	4	5
Gold Medal Ribbon	1	170	19	0	19	3	8
Jamoca Almond Fudge	1	170	17	1	16	3	9
Lemon Sorbet	1	80	21	0	21	0	0
Mango Fruit Blast smoothie	16 oz.	440	104	2	102	4	2
Mango Sorbet	1	80	20	0	20	0	0
Milk Chocolate, light churned	1	130	20	1	19	4	5
Mint Chocolate Chip	1	170	15	0	15	3	10
Mint *Oreo*, light churned	1	150	25	1	24	3	5
Old Fashioned Butter Pecan	1	170	20	1	19	3	11
Orange Sherbet Freeze	16 oz.	370	82	0	82	3	4
Oreo Cookies 'n Cream	1	170	15	0	15	3	9
Peach Passion Banana Fruit Blast smoothie	16 oz.	420	102	4	98	6	1
Peach Passion Fruit Blast	16 oz.	270	68	2	66	1	0
Pineapple Coconut, reduced fat, no sugar added	1	100	18	2	16	3	4

	SERVING SIZE	CALORIES	TOTAL CARBS (g)	FIBER (g)	NET CARBS (g)	PROTEIN (g)	FAT (g)
Baskin Robbins (cont.)	. . .	. . .	.	.	.	.	.
Pistachio Almond	1	180	22	1	21	4	12
Pralines and Cream	1	180	19	0	19	3	9
Rainbow sherbet	1	100	21	0	21	1	1.5
Raspberry Chip, light churned	1	140	24	1	23	3	4
Reese's Peanut Butter Cup	1	190	19	0	19	4	11
Rocky road ice cream	1	180	22	0	22	3	10
Strawberry Banana Fruit Blast smoothie	16 oz.	390	94	3	91	5	Tr
Strawberry Citrus Fruit Blast	16 oz.	240	61	1	60	1	0
Strawberry Sorbet	1	80	21	0	21	0	0
Sugar Cone	1	45	9	0	9	1	Tr
Vanilla ice cream	1	170	17	0	17	3	10
Vanilla yogurt, Fat-Free	1	90	20	0	20	4	0
Vanilla, light churned	1	130	19	1	18	4	5
Very Berry Strawberry	1	140	18	0	18	2	7
Waffle Cone	1	160	28	0	28	2	4
Wild Mango Fruit Blast	16 oz.	340	84	2	82	1	1
World Class Chocolate	1	180	19	0	19	3	10
Blimpie	*(all subs on a 6" regular roll unless otherwise stated)*	. . .	.	.	.	.	.
Antipasto salad	1	250	12	4	8	20	14

	SERVING SIZE	CALORIES	TOTAL CARBS (g)	FIBER (g)	NET CARBS (g)	PROTEIN (g)	FAT (g)
Blimpie (cont.)	...	...	.	.	.	.	.
Apple turnover	1	340	35	1	34	4	21
Bacon, egg & cheese biscuit	1	430	37	1	36	17	24
Bacon, egg & cheese bluffin	1	290	27	2	25	16	14
Bacon, egg & cheese burrito	1	550	56	5	51	31	24
Bacon, egg & cheese croissant	1	400	30	1	29	16	115
Bean w/ ham soup	1	140	23	11	12	8	1
Beef steak & noodle soup	1	120	14	0	14	8	3
Beef stew	1	170	18	2	16	17	4
Biscuit, plain	1	260	34	1	33	6	11
Blimpie best	1	420	49	3	46	25	14
Blimpie best, super stacked	1	520	52	3	49	37	19
Blimpie trio, super stacked	1	490	52	3	49	41	12
BLT	1	450	46	3	43	15	22
BLT, super stacked	1	640	43	2	41	22	41
Blue cheese dressing	1.5 oz	230	2	Tr	2	2	24
Bluffin, plain	1	30	25	2	23	5	1
Breakfast panini, 4"	1	490	67	2	65	26	14
Breakfast panini, 6"	1	770	96	3	93	43	24
Brownie	1	180	28	1	27	2	7
Buffalo chicken ciabatta	1	580	50	3	47	32	27
Buffalo chicken salad	1	220	10	4	6	25	9
Buttermilk ranch dressing	1.5 oz	230	2	Tr	2	1	24
Captain's corn chowder	1	210	29	4	25	6	7

	SERVING SIZE	CALORIES	TOTAL CARBS (g)	FIBER (g)	NET CARBS (g)	PROTEIN (g)	FAT (g)
Blimple (cont.)	. . .	. . .	.	.	.	.	.
Chef salad	1	180	10	2	8	18	7
Cherry turnover	1	350	35	1	34	4	21
Chicken & dumpling soup	1	170	19	3	16	11	5
Chicken caesar salad	1	190	6	3	3	25	8
Chicken caesar wrap	1	610	56	4	52	30	29
Chicken cheddar bacon ranch	1	640	48	3	45	36	34
Chicken gumbo	1	90	13	2	11	6	2
Chicken noodle soup	1	130	18	2	16	7	4
Chicken teriyaki	1	430	50	1	49	35	9
Chicken teriyaki, on wheat	1	420	47	5	42	36	10
Chicken w/ white & wild rice soup	1	250	15	4	11	14	10
Chocolate chunk cookie	1	200	25	0	25	2	10
Cinnamon roll	1	450	60	2	58	9	20
Club	1	390	49	3	46	25	10
Club, on wheat	1	360	43	6	37	26	11
Cole slaw	1 svg	160	20	2	18	1	9
Cream of broccoli w/ cheese soup	1	190	15	3	12	6	8
Cream of potato soup	1	190	24	3	21	5	9
Creamy caesar dressing	1.5 oz	210	2	Tr	2	1	21
Creamy italian dressing	1.5 oz	180	4	0	4	0	18
Croissant, plain	1	230	28	1	27	5	102
Cuban	1	410	43	1	42	29	11

	SERVING SIZE	CALORIES	TOTAL CARBS (g)	FIBER (g)	NET CARBS (g)	PROTEIN (g)	FAT (g)
Blimpie (cont.)	...	...	.	.	.	.	.
Deli style mustard	0.5 oz	5	0	0	0	0	0
Dijon honey mustard dressing	1.5 oz	180	8	Tr	8	1	17
Egg & cheese biscuit	1	390	37	1	36	14	21
Egg & cheese bluffin	1	250	27	2	25	13	10
Egg & cheese burrito	1	510	56	5	51	28	20
Egg & cheese croissant	1	350	30	1	29	12	111
Fat-free italian dressing	1.5 oz	25	5	0	5	0	0
French dip	1	410	46	1	45	30	11
French onion soup	1	80	11	1	10	2	4
Garden salad	1	30	6	3	3	2	0
Grande chili w/ bean & beef	1	250	30	18	12	18	9
Grilled chicken caesar ciabatta	1	620	63	3	60	34	24
Ham & swiss	1	390	50	3	47	25	10
Ham & swiss, on wheat	1	370	44	6	38	26	11
Ham, egg & cheese biscuit	1	420	39	1	38	19	21
Ham, egg & cheese bluffin	1	280	29	2	27	18	11
Ham, egg & cheese burrito	1	560	58	5	53	36	21
Ham, egg & cheese croissant	1	380	31	1	30	17	112
Ham, salami & cheese	1	440	49	3	46	25	16
Harvest vegetable soup	1	100	19	3	16	4	1

	SERVING SIZE	CALORIES	TOTAL CARBS (g)	FIBER (g)	NET CARBS (g)	PROTEIN (g)	FAT (g)
Blimpie (cont.)	...	...	.	.	.	.	.
Honey mustard	1 oz	45	7	1	6	1	1
Hot pastrami	1	440	42	1	41	30	16
Hot pastrami, super stacked	1	570	43	1	42	46	23
Italian style wedding soup	1	130	17	0	17	7	4
Light buttermilk ranch dressing	1.5 oz	70	8	Tr	8	1	4
Light italian dressing	1.5 oz	20	2	Tr	2	0	1
Macaroni salad	1 svg	330	28	2	26	5	22
Mayonnaise	1 oz	200	0	0	0	0	22
Meatball	1	600	51	4	47	28	32
Mediterranean ciabatta	1	450	65	3	62	26	8
Minestrone	1	90	14	4	10	4	3
New England clam chowder	1	170	28	2	26	7	3
Northwest potato salad	1 svg	260	22	3	19	3	17
Oatmeal raisin cookie	1	170	26	1	25	2	7
Oil blend	0.5 oz	130	0	0	0	0	14
Pasta fagioli w/ sausage	1	150	22	4	18	7	5
Peanut butter cookie	1	200	20	1	19	3	12
Peppercorn dressing	1.5 oz	240	1	0	1	1	26
Philly steak & onion	1	500	45	1	44	26	24
Pilgrim turkey vegetables w/ rice soup	1	110	19	2	17	4	2
Potato salad	1 svg	230	28	3	25	3	12
Red hot original sauce	1 oz	10	2	0	2	0	0

	SERVING SIZE	CALORIES	TOTAL CARBS (g)	FIBER (g)	NET CARBS (g)	PROTEIN (g)	FAT (g)
Blimple (cont.)	...	...	.	.	.	.	.
Red wine vinegar	0.5 oz	5	1	0	1	0	0
Reuben	1	570	54	3	51	34	24
Roast beef & cheddar wrap	1	680	59	6	53	32	36
Roast beef & provolone	1	410	47	3	44	31	11
Roast beef & provolone, on wheat	1	390	40	6	34	32	12
Roast beef, turkey & cheddar	1	570	48	3	45	27	30
Roast beef, turkey & cheddar ciabatta	1	590	51	3	48	28	30
Sausage, egg & cheese biscuit	1	540	37	1	36	20	35
Sausage, egg & cheese bluffin	1	400	27	2	25	19	24
Sausage, egg & cheese burrito	1	660	56	5	51	34	34
Sausage, egg, & cheese croissant	1	500	30	1	29	18	125
Seafood	1	330	56	4	52	13	7
Seafood gumbo	1	100	16	2	14	4	2
Seafood salad	1	120	17	3	14	6	4
Sicilian ciabatta	1	640	68	3	65	33	25
Southwestern wrap	1	530	61	4	57	23	22
Special dressing	0.7 oz	70	0	Tr	0	0	7
Special vegetarian	1	590	66	4	62	17	30
Spicy brown mustard	0.5 oz	5	0	Tr	0	0	0
Split pea w/ ham soup	1	130	21	6	15	8	2
Steak & onion wrap	1	770	62	6	56	28	47
Sugar cookie	1	330	41	1	40	3	17

	SERVING SIZE	CALORIES	TOTAL CARBS (g)	FIBER (g)	NET CARBS (g)	PROTEIN (g)	FAT (g)
Blimpie (cont.)	...	...	.	.	.	.	.
Thousand island dressing	1.5 oz	210	6	0	6	0	20
Tomato basil w/ raviolini soup	1	110	22	0	22	4	1
Tuna	1	480	46	3	43	25	21
Tuna salad	1	270	7	2	5	18	18
Turkey & avocado	1	380	52	4	48	21	9
Turkey & bacon, super stacked	1	580	48	2	46	40	24
Turkey & cranberry	1	350	58	3	55	20	4
Turkey & provolone	1	390	49	3	46	26	10
Turkey & provolone, on wheat	1	370	43	6	37	27	10
Turkey italiano ciabatta	1	500	64	3	61	30	11
Tuscan ciabatta	1	600	65	3	62	29	23
Ultimate club ciabatta	1	480	47	2	45	27	21
Ultimate club salad	1	290	10	3	7	25	16
Veggie supreme	1	550	48	3	45	29	28
Vegimax	1	520	56	5	51	28	20
Vegimax, on wheat	1	500	50	8	42	30	21
White chocolate macadamia nut cookie	1	200	20	1	19	3	12
Yankee pot roast soup	1	80	12	2	10	5	2
Zesty wrap	1	570	59	6	53	28	26
Boston Market	...	...	.	.	.	.	.
Apple pie	1 slice	580	74	3	71	43	30
Baked beans	1 svg	270	53	11	42	11	2
BBQ brisket meal	1	400	28	0	28	26	20
BBQ brisket sandwich	1	800	90	3	87	43	30

	SERVING SIZE	CALORIES	TOTAL CARBS (g)	FIBER (g)	NET CARBS (g)	PROTEIN (g)	FAT (g)
Boston Market (cont.)	...	...	.	.	.	.	.
BBQ chicken, half	1	730	28	1	27	90	30
BBQ dark chicken	3 pc	430	28	1	27	52	13
Beef brisket meal	1	280	1	0	1	26	20
Beef gravy	3 oz	35	4	0	4	1	2
Boston chicken carver sandwich	1	750	64	3	61	57	29
Boston chicken carver sandwich, half	1	375	32	1	31	28	15
Boston meatloaf carver sandwich	1	980	92	4	88	47	46
Boston turkey carver sandwich	1	700	65	3	62	50	26
Boston turkey carver sandwich, half	1	350	32	2	30	25	13
Brisket dip carver sandwich	1	890	63	3	60	43	51
Caesar salad dressing	2.5 oz	360	4	1	3	2	38
Caesar salad entrée	1	420	9	2	7	12	38
Caesar side salad	1	180	4	1	3	4	17
Chicken noodle soup	1	250	23	2	21	22	8
Chicken tortilla soup	1	410	30	2	28	17	26
Chocolate cake	1 svg	580	67	3	64	5	34
Chocolate chip fudge brownie	1	320	49	3	46	5	13
Cinnamon apples	1 svg	210	47	3	44	0	3
Classic chicken salad sandwich	1	800	65	4	61	40	41
Coleslaw	1 svg	300	27	4	23	2	20
Cornbread	1 svg	180	31	0	31	2	5

	SERVING SIZE	CALORIES	TOTAL CARBS (g)	FIBER (g)	NET CARBS (g)	PROTEIN (g)	FAT (g)
***Boston Market** (cont.)*	. . .	. . .	.	.	.	.	.
Creamed spinach	1 svg	280	12	4	8	9	23
Crispy country chicken carver sandwich	1	1020	114	4	110	45	42
Crispy country chicken w/ country gravy	1	480	36	1	35	33	23
Crispy country chicken, add on	3 oz	220	16	1	15	16	11
Dark individual meal	3 pc	390	1	0	1	51	22
Dark individual meal, 2 thighs & drumstick	3 pc	490	0	0	0	60	29
Dark skinless meal, 2 thighs & drumstick	3 pc	350	0	0	0	52	15
Dark skinless meal, thigh & 2 drumsticks	3 pc	290	0	0	0	45	11
Fresh steamed vegetables	1 svg	60	8	3	5	2	2
Fresh vegetable stuffing	1 svg	190	25	2	23	3	8
Fruit salad	1 svg	60	15	1	14	1	0
Garlic dill new potatoes	1 svg	140	24	3	21	3	3
Green beans	1 svg	60	7	3	4	2	4
Lite ranch dressing	1.5 oz	70	8	0	8	1	4
Macaroni & cheese	1 svg	300	35	2	33	11	11
Market chopped salad	1	480	24	7	17	9	40
Market chopped salad dressing	2.5 oz	360	2	0	2	0	39
Mashed potatoes	1 svg	270	36	4	32	5	11

	SERVING SIZE	CALORIES	TOTAL CARBS (g)	FIBER (g)	NET CARBS (g)	PROTEIN (g)	FAT (g)
Boston Market (cont.)	...	...	.	.	.	.	.
Meatloaf meal	1	520	21	0	21	29	36
Meatloaf open-faced sandwich	1	670	48	1	47	34	38
Pastry top chicken pot pie	1	800	59	4	55	32	48
Potato salad	1 svg	390	26	3	23	3	29
Poultry gravy	4 oz	50	7	0	7	0	2
Roasted sirloin open-faced sandwich	1	410	32	1	31	35	15
Roasted sirloin, add on	3 oz	160	0	0	0	26	6
Roasted turkey meal	1	150	0	0	0	31	3
Roasted turkey open-faced sandwich	1	330	43	1	42	26	6
Roasted turkey, add on	3 oz	110	0	0	0	23	2
Rotisserie chicken open-faced sandwich	1	320	34	1	33	27	8
Rotisserie chicken, add on	5 oz	180	0	0	0	39	3
Rotisserie chicken, half	1	610	1	0	1	89	29
Smokehouse BBQ chicken sandwich	1	850	101	4	97	44	29
Sweet corn	1 svg	170	37	2	35	6	4
Sweet potato casserole	1 svg	460	77	3	74	4	16
Thigh & drumstick	1	290	0	0	0	37	17
White BBQ Chicken, quarter	1	430	28	1	27	52	13
White rotisserie chicken, no skin, quarter	1	240	1	0	1	50	4

	SERVING SIZE	CALORIES	TOTAL CARBS (g)	FIBER (g)	NET CARBS (g)	PROTEIN (g)	FAT (g)
Boston Market (cont.)	. . .	. . .	.	.	.	.	.
White rotisserie chicken, quarter	1	320	0	0	0	52	12
Bruegger's	*(all sandwiches on plain bagel, unless otherwise stated)*	. . .	.	.	.	.	.
Asiago parmesan bagel	1	330	61	4	57	14	20
Asian sesame ginger dressing	2 oz	260	17	0	17	0	21
Bacon scallion cream cheese	1	140	5	0	5	3	12
Balsamic vinaigrette dressing	2 oz	110	8	0	8	0	9
Beef chili	1	190	18	6	12	10	8
BLT	1	570	72	5	67	20	23
Blueberry bagel	1	320	67	4	63	11	2
Blueberry muffin	1	400	57	2	55	7	17
Breakfast bagel sandwich w/ ham	1	460	73	4	69	31	18
Breakfast bagel sandwich w/ sausage	1	640	63	4	59	29	30
Breakfast bagel sandwich, no meat	1	420	71	4	67	23	18
Breakfast bagel sandwich w/ bacon	1	460	65	4	61	28	23
Butternut squash soup	1	240	21	1	20	4	17
Caesar dressing	2 oz	110	8	0	8	2	9
Caesar salad w/ chicken & dressing	1	380	23	2	21	28	20

	SERVING SIZE	CALORIES	TOTAL CARBS (g)	FIBER (g)	NET CARBS (g)	PROTEIN (g)	FAT (g)
Bruegger's (cont.)	...	...	.	.	.	.	.
Caesar salad w/ dressing	1	270	22	2	20	9	17
Caesar salad, no dressing	1	160	14	2	12	7	8
Chicken breast sandwich	1	660	87	5	82	47	11
Chicken spaetzle soup	1	140	15	1	14	8	5
Chicken wild rice soup	1	280	12	1	11	8	22
Chocolate chip bagel	1	350	64	4	60	12	5
Chocolate chip cookie	1	390	52	2	50	5	17
Chocolate chunk brownie	1	330	40	2	38	4	18
Chocolate muffin	1	460	57	3	54	6	24
Cinnamon raisin bagel	1	330	69	4	65	11	2
Cinnamon sugar bagel	1	350	73	6	67	12	2
Classic wrap w/ bacon	1	520	52	4	48	36	45
Classic wrap w/ ham	1	510	54	4	50	40	41
Classic wrap w/ sausage	1	590	15	4	11	35	53
Cranberry orange bagel	1	330	68	4	64	11	2
Double chocolate cookie	1	390	51	3	48	5	19
Everything bagel	1	310	31	4	27	12	2
Everything cookie	1	380	49	2	47	5	18
Fire roasted tomato soup	1	130	17	2	15	2	6

	SERVING SIZE	CALORIES	TOTAL CARBS (g)	FIBER (g)	NET CARBS (g)	PROTEIN (g)	FAT (g)
Bruegger's (cont.)	. . .	. . .	.	.	.	.	.
Fortified multigrain bagel	1	350	69	6	63	13	4
Four cheese & tomato panini on hearty white	1	700	57	3	54	42	35
Four cheese broccoli soup	1	260	12	1	11	9	20
Garden veggie cream cheese	1	130	5	1	4	3	11
Garden veggie sandwich	1	400	82	7	75	16	3
Garlic bagel	1	320	65	4	61	12	2
Ham & swiss Panini on honey wheat	1	600	71	2	69	39	18
Ham sandwich	1	410	66	4	62	27	5
Herby turkey sandwich on sesame bagel	1	600	80	5	75	43	14
Honey grain bagel	1	330	65	5	60	13	3
Honey walnut cream cheese	1	150	8	Tr	8	3	12
Jalapeno bagel	1	320	64	4	60	12	2
Jalapeno cream cheese	1	140	4	0	4	3	13
Leonardo da veggie sandwich on asiago softwich	1	590	83	7	76	28	17
Light garden veggie cream cheese	1	90	3	0	3	6	6
Light herb garlic cream cheese	1	100	4	0	4	6	6
Light plain cream cheese	1	100	4	Tr	4	6	6
Mandarin medley salad w/ balsamic vinaigrette	1	340	36	4	32	8	17

	SERVING SIZE	CALORIES	TOTAL CARBS (g)	FIBER (g)	NET CARBS (g)	PROTEIN (g)	FAT (g)
Bruegger's (cont.)	. . .	. . .	.	.	.	.	.
Mandarin medley salad w/ chicken & balsamic vinaigrette	1	450	37	4	33	26	21
Mandarin medley salad, no dressing	1	230	29	4	25	8	8
Marshmallow chew bar	1	280	55	0	55	2	6
New England clam chowder	1	230	16	Tr	16	23	14
Olive pimiento cream cheese	1	140	3	0	3	3	13
Onion & chive cream cheese	1	140	3	0	3	3	13
Onion bagel	1	320	64	4	60	12	2
Plain bagel	1	300	60	4	56	12	2
Plain cream cheese	1	130	6	Tr	6	3	11
Poppy bagel	1	310	61	4	57	12	3
Primo pesto chicken panini on hearty white	1	700	56	2	54	49	32
Pumpernickel bagel	1	330	67	5	62	12	3
Ranch dressing	2 oz	190	2	0	2	0	21
Rio Grande wrap w/ bacon	1	560	55	4	51	34	49
Rio Grande wrap w/ ham	1	630	55	4	51	31	34
Rio Grande wrap w/ sausage	1	510	53	4	49	27	47
Roast beef sandwich	1	730	71	5	66	30	39
Roma roast beef sandwich on hearty white	1	770	62	3	59	46	44

	SERVING SIZE	CALORIES	TOTAL CARBS (g)	FIBER (g)	NET CARBS (g)	PROTEIN (g)	FAT (g)
Bruegger's (cont.)	...	...	.	.	.	.	.
Rosemary olive oil bagel	1	350	64	4	60	12	7
Sesame bagel	1	310	61	4	57	13	3
Sesame salad w/ asian sesame dressing	1	380	29	2	27	23	26
Sesame salad w/ chicken & asian sesame dressing	1	490	30	2	28	42	29
Sesame salad, no dressing	1	120	12	2	10	4	5
Seven layer bar	1	650	58	5	53	10	43
Smoked salmon cream cheese	1	150	3	Tr	3	3	13
Smoked salmon sandwich	1	460	65	5	60	27	10
Sourdough bagel	1	310	63	4	59	12	2
Spinach & cheddar omelet sandwich	1	500	64	4	60	24	16
Spinach & lentil soup	1	110	16	7	9	7	4
Spinach, cheddar & bacon omelet, on sesame bagel	1	550	60	3	57	28	22
Spinach, cheddar & ham omelet, on sesame bagel	1	540	65	4	61	30	17
Spinach, cheddar & sausage omelet, on sesame bagel	1	660	64	4	60	29	32
Strawberry cream cheese	1	140	4	0	4	3	13

	SERVING SIZE	CALORIES	TOTAL CARBS (g)	FIBER (g)	NET CARBS (g)	PROTEIN (g)	FAT (g)
Bruegger's (cont.)	...	...	.	.	.	.	.
Sundried tomato bagel	1	320	64	4	60	12	2
Tarragon chicken salad sandwich on hearty white	1	770	73	3	70	59	41
Thai peanut chicken sandwich	1	580	91	7	84	28	11
Toffee almond bar	1	400	53	1	52	4	19
Tuna & cheddar melt on honey wheat	1	1020	61	3	58	42	67
Tuna salad sandwich	1	620	73	5	68	23	27
Turkey chipotle club on honey wheat	1	800	57	3	54	31	51
Turkey sandwich	1	510	70	5	65	26	14
Turkey toscana Panini on hearty white	1	710	59	3	56	41	37
Western omelet sandwich	1	760	66	4	62	27	56
White chicken chili	1	240	26	7	19	14	9
Whole wheat bagel	1	390	73	9	64	22	6
Burger King	...	...	.	.	.	.	.
Bacon, egg & cheese biscuit	1	430	34	1	33	17	25
Barbecue dipping sauce	1 oz	40	11	0	11	0	0
BK Big Fish sandwich	1	640	66	3	63	23	32
BK Breakfast Shots, bacon & cheese, 2 pack	1	310	18	1	17	14	20

	SERVING SIZE	CALORIES	TOTAL CARBS (g)	FIBER (g)	NET CARBS (g)	PROTEIN (g)	FAT (g)
Burger King (cont.)	. . .	. . .	.	.	.	.	.
BK Breakfast Shots, ham & cheese, 2 pack	1	270	18	1	17	13	16
BK Breakfast Shots, sausage & cheese, 2 pack	1	420	18	1	17	18	31
BK Burger Shot, 2 pack	1	220	18	1	17	14	10
BK Burger Shots, 6 pack	1	650	53	2	51	40	31
BK Chicken fries, 12 pieces/svg	1 svg	500	32	3	29	28	29
BK Chicken fries, 6 pieces/svg	1 svg	250	16	1	15	14	15
BK Chicken fries, 9 pieces/svg	1 svg	380	24	2	22	21	22
BK Double Stacker	1	620	32	1	31	34	39
BK Fresh Apple fries	1 svg	25	6	1	5	0	0
BK Quad Stacker	1	1010	34	1	33	64	70
BK Triple Stacker	1	820	33	1	32	49	55
BK Veggie burger	1	420	46	7	39	23	16
BK Veggie burger w/ cheese	1	470	47	7	40	25	20
Breakfast syrup	1 svg	80	21	0	21	0	0
Buffalo dipping sauce	1 oz	80	2	0	2	1	8
Caramel sauce	1 svg	45	10	0	10	0	Tr
Cheeseburger	1	340	31	1	30	18	16
Cheesy Bacon BK Wrapper	1	390	29	2	27	14	24
Cheesy Tots potatoes, 12 pieces/svg	1 svg	440	41	4	37	14	24

	SERVING SIZE	CALORIES	TOTAL CARBS (g)	FIBER (g)	NET CARBS (g)	PROTEIN (g)	FAT (g)
Burger King (cont.)	...	...	.	.	.	.	.
Cheesy Tots potatoes, 6 pieces/svg	1 svg	220	21	2	19	7	12
Cheesy Tots potatoes, 9 pieces/svg	1 svg	330	31	3	28	11	18
Chicken sandwich, original	1	630	46	3	43	24	39
Chicken tenders, 4 pieces/svg	1 svg	180	13	0	13	9	11
Chicken tenders, 5 pieces/svg	1 svg	230	16	0	16	11	13
Chicken tenders, 6 pieces/svg	1 svg	270	19	0	19	14	16
Chicken tenders, 8 pieces/svg	1 svg	360	25	0	25	18	21
Chocolate milk shake, sm	12 fl oz	310	53	1	52	6	11
Cini-minis, 4 pieces	1 svg	400	52	2	50	7	18
Cini-minis, 4 pieces, w/ vanilla icing	1 svg	490	74	2	72	7	18
Croissan'wich w/ bacon, egg & cheese	1	350	27	0	27	15	19
Croissan'wich w/ egg & cheese	1	310	27	0	27	12	16
Croissan'wich w/ ham, egg & cheese	1	340	28	0	28	18	17
Croissan'wich w/ sausage & cheese	1	380	26	0	26	14	24

	SERVING SIZE	CALORIES	TOTAL CARBS (g)	FIBER (g)	NET CARBS (g)	PROTEIN (g)	FAT (g)
Burger King (cont.)	...	...	.	.	.	.	.
Croissan'wich w/ sausage, egg & cheese	1	470	28	0	28	20	31
Double cheeseburger	1	510	31	1	30	30	29
Double Croissan'wich w/ bacon, egg & cheese	1	430	28	0	28	20	26
Double Croissan'wich w/ ham, bacon, egg & cheese	1	430	29	0	29	23	24
Double Croissan'wich w/ ham, egg & cheese	1	420	30	0	30	26	21
Double Croissan'wich w/ ham, sausage, egg & cheese	1	550	30	0	30	28	36
Double Croissan'wich w/ sausage, bacon, egg & cheese	1	560	29	0	29	25	38
Double Croissan'wich w/ sausage, egg & cheese	1	690	30	0	30	30	50
Double hamburger	1	420	30	1	29	26	22
Double whopper	1	920	51	3	48	48	58
Double whopper w/ cheese	1	1010	53	3	50	53	66
Dutch apple pie	1	320	47	1	46	2	13

	SERVING SIZE	CALORIES	TOTAL CARBS (g)	FIBER (g)	NET CARBS (g)	PROTEIN (g)	FAT (g)
Burger King (cont.)	...	...	.	.	.	.	.
French fries, large	1 svg	580	74	6	68	6	28
French fries, med	1 svg	480	61	5	56	5	23
French fries, small	1 svg	340	44	4	40	4	17
French fries, value	1 svg	220	28	2	26	2	11
French toast sticks, 3 pieces/svg	1 svg	230	29	1	28	3	11
French toast sticks, 5 pieces/svg	1 svg	380	49	2	47	5	18
Garden salad w/o dressing	1	70	7	3	4	4	4
Garlic Parmesan Croutons	1 svg	60	9	0	9	1	2
Ham omelet sandwich	1	290	33	1	32	13	12
Ham, egg & cheese biscuit	1	410	34	1	33	17	23
Hamburger	1	290	30	1	29	15	12
Hash browns, medium	1	610	58	8	50	5	39
Hash browns, small	1	420	40	6	34	3	27
Hash browns, value size	1	250	24	3	21	2	16
Hershey's Sundae Pie	1	310	32	1	31	3	19
Honey mustard dipping sauce	1 oz	90	8	0	8	7	6
Jam, strawberry or grape	1 svg	30	7	0	7	0	0
Ken's Creamy Caesar dressing	2 oz	210	4	0	4	3	21
Ken's Honey Mustard dressing	2 oz	270	15	0	15	1	23

	SERVING SIZE	CALORIES	TOTAL CARBS (g)	FIBER (g)	NET CARBS (g)	PROTEIN (g)	FAT (g)
Burger King (cont.)	. . .	. . .	.	.	.	.	.
Ken's Light Italian dressing	2 oz	120	5	0	5	0	11
Ken's Ranch dressing	2 oz	190	2	0	2	1	20
Ketchup	1 pkt	10	3	0	3	0	0
Kraft Macaroni & Cheese	1 svg	160	22	1	21	7	5
Mayonnaise	1 pkt	80	1	0	1	0	9
Mushroom & Swiss Steakhouse XT	1	870	54	4	50	43	49
Onion rings, large	1 svg	510	60	5	55	7	27
Onion rings, medium	1 svg	450	52	5	47	6	24
Onion rings, small	1 svg	310	36	3	33	4	17
Onion rings, value size	1 svg	150	17	1	16	2	8
Oreo BK Sundae Shake, chocolate, sm	16 fl oz	700	116	2	114	11	26
Oreo BK Sundae Shake, strawberry, sm	16 fl oz	680	114	1	113	10	25
Ranch dipping sauce	1 oz	140	1	0	1	1	15
Sausage biscuit	1	420	32	1	31	13	27
Sausage, egg & Cheese biscuit	1	560	35	1	34	21	37
Spicy Chick'n Crisp sandwich	1	450	34	2	32	12	30
Steakhouse Burger	1	950	55	4	51	40	59
Steakhouse XT	1	970	55	4	51	42	61
Strawberry milk shake, sm	12 fl oz	310	52	0	52	6	11

	SERVING SIZE	CALORIES	TOTAL CARBS (g)	FIBER (g)	NET CARBS (g)	PROTEIN (g)	FAT (g)
Burger King (cont.)	...	...	.	.	.	.	.
Sweet & sour dipping sauce	1 oz	45	11	0	11	0	0
Tendercrisp Chicken garden salad	1	410	27	4	23	27	23
Tendercrisp Chicken sandwich	1	800	68	3	65	32	46
Tendergrill Chicken garden salad	1	210	8	3	5	29	7
Tendergrill Chicken sandwich	1	490	51	3	48	26	21
Three Cheese Steakhouse XT	1	1050	52	3	49	51	71
Triple Whopper	1	1160	51	3	48	68	76
Triple Whopper w/ cheese	1	1250	52	3	49	73	84
Vanilla milk shake, sm	12 fl oz	270	42	0	42	6	11
Whopper	1	670	51	3	48	29	40
Whopper junior	1	370	31	2	29	16	21
Whopper junior w/ cheese	1	420	31	2	29	18	25
Whopper w/ cheese	1	770	52	3	49	33	48
Zesty onion ring dipping sauce	1 oz	150	3	1	2	0	15
Carl's Jr.	...	...	.	.	.	.	.
Bacon & egg burrito	1	550	37	1	36	29	32
Bacon Swiss Crispy Chicken sandwich	1	750	62	4	58	36	40
Big hamburger	1	460	54	3	51	24	17
Blue cheese dressing	2 oz	320	1	0	1	2	34

	SERVING SIZE	CALORIES	TOTAL CARBS (g)	FIBER (g)	NET CARBS (g)	PROTEIN (g)	FAT (g)
Carl's Jr. (cont.)	...	...	.	.	.	.	.
Breakfast Burger	1	780	64	3	61	38	41
Carl's Catch fish sandwich	1	710	74	4	70	20	37
Charbroiled BBQ Chicken sandwich	1	380	49	2	47	34	7
Charbroiled Chicken Club sandwich	1	560	44	2	42	39	27
Charbroiled chicken salad	1	250	14	4	10	29	9
Charbroiled Santa Fe Chicken sandwich	1	630	44	2	42	36	35
Chicken Stars	4 pc	210	10	1	9	8	16
Chicken Stars	6 pc	320	14	2	12	12	24
Chicken Stars	9 pc	480	21	2	19	18	36
Chicken strips	3 pc	370	19	2	17	14	26
Chicken strips	5 pc	610	32	3	29	23	43
Chili cheese fries	1 svg	990	89	8	81	28	56
Chili cheeseburger	1	780	58	4	54	41	41
Chocolate cake	1 pc	300	48	1	47	3	12
Chocolate chip cookie	1	370	48	2	46	3	19
Chocolate malt	1	780	100	1	99	15	34
Chocolate shake	1	710	86	1	85	14	33
CrissCut fries	1 svg	450	42	4	38	5	29
Double Western Bacon Cheeseburger	1	960	70	3	67	52	52
Famous Star w/ cheese	1	660	53	3	50	27	39
Fish & chips	1 svg	730	72	6	66	22	39

	SERVING SIZE	CALORIES	TOTAL CARBS (g)	FIBER (g)	NET CARBS (g)	PROTEIN (g)	FAT (g)
Carl's Jr. (cont.)	...	...	.	.	.	.	.
French Toast Dips, no syrup	5 pc	460	60	3	57	9	21
Fried zucchini	1 svg	330	36	2	34	6	18
Green Burrito taco salad	1	970	76	17	59	42	58
Hash brown nuggets	1 svg	350	32	3	29	3	23
House dressing	2 oz	220	3	0	3	1	22
Jalapeno Burger	1	720	50	3	47	27	46
Loaded breakfast burrito	1	780	51	3	48	36	49
Low fat balsamic dressing	2 oz	35	5	0	5	0	2
Natural-cut fries, large	1	500	65	5	60	6	24
Natural-cut fries, medium	1	460	60	5	55	5	22
Natural-cut fries, small	1	320	42	4	38	4	15
Onion rings	1 svg	530	61	3	58	8	28
Oreo cookie malt	1	790	95	1	94	17	38
Oreo cookie shake	1	730	81	1	80	15	38
Side salad	1	50	4	2	2	3	3
Sourdough breakfast sandwich	1	450	38	1	37	29	21
Spicy chicken sandwich	1	420	33	2	31	12	27
Steak & egg burrito	1	650	43	1	42	41	36
Strawberry malt	1	770	99	0	99	15	34
Strawberry shake	1	700	85	0	85	14	33
Strawberry swirl cheesecake	1 pc	290	32	0	32	6	16

	SERVING SIZE	CALORIES	TOTAL CARBS (g)	FIBER (g)	NET CARBS (g)	PROTEIN (g)	FAT (g)
Carl's Jr. (cont.)	...	...	.	.	.	.	.
Sunrise Croissant sandwich	1	590	27	1	26	20	44
Super Star w/ cheese	1	920	54	3	51	47	58
The Bacon Cheese Six Dollar Burger	1	950	49	3	46	51	62
The Guacamole Bacon Six Dollar Burger	1	1040	53	4	49	49	70
The Jalapeno Six Dollar Burger	1	930	52	3	49	45	61
The Low Carb Six Dollar Burger	1	570	7	1	6	38	43
The Original Six Dollar Burger	1	890	58	3	55	45	54
The Western Bacon Six Dollar Burger	1	1020	81	3	78	53	53
Thousand island dressing	2 oz	240	7	0	7	0	23
Vanilla malt	1	780	101	0	101	15	34
Vanilla shake	1	710	86	0	86	14	33
Western Bacon Cheeseburger	1	710	69	3	66	32	33
Checkers	...	...	.	.	.	.	.
All beef hot dog	1	280	23	2	21	11	17
Bacon Buford	1	680	31	3	28	34	46
Bacon cheddar burger	1	370	29	2	27	20	19
Bacon cheddar fries	1	560	44	5	39	11	37
Bacon double bacon	1	710	43	3	40	38	43
Bacon double cheeseburger	1	650	32	4	28	35	42

	SERVING SIZE	CALORIES	TOTAL CARBS (g)	FIBER (g)	NET CARBS (g)	PROTEIN (g)	FAT (g)
Checkers (cont.)	...	...	.	.	.	.	.
Bacon philly cheesesteak burger	1	560	42	2	40	31	30
Bacon ranch fries	1	640	50	5	45	12	43
Bacon Swiss Buford	1	660	28	4	24	35	45
Banana shake, medium	1	440	71	0	71	11	12
Big Buford	1	570	31	3	28	31	36
BLT	1	380	47	4	43	13	16
Checkerburger	1	390	32	3	29	16	22
Checkerburger w/ cheese	1	420	33	3	30	18	24
Cheese double cheese	1	510	31	3	28	29	31
Chili cheese dog	1	390	28	3	25	17	23
Chili cheese fries	1	550	48	6	42	13	34
Chili cheeseburger	1	320	30	3	27	18	15
Chili dog	1	410	27	3	24	19	25
Chocolate shake, medium	1	430	72	0	72	9	12
Cinnamon apple pie	1	240	31	2	29	3	12
Crispy chicken breast sandwich	1	610	61	4	57	26	29
Crispy chicken club sandwich	1	740	60	4	56	34	41
Crispy fish sandwich	1	430	51	4	47	14	19
Deep Sea Double	1	640	63	5	58	25	31
Double chili cheeseburger	1	460	30	3	27	27	26
Double decker	1	480	31	3	28	27	28

	SERVING SIZE	CALORIES	TOTAL CARBS (g)	FIBER (g)	NET CARBS (g)	PROTEIN (g)	FAT (g)
Checkers (cont.)	. . .	. . .	.	.	.	.	.
Frank's Red Hot chicken sandwich	1	340	34	2	32	16	16
Fries, large	1	590	57	6	51	7	38
Fries, medium	1	420	40	4	36	5	27
Fries, small	1	300	28	3	25	3	19
Fully loaded bacon cheddar ranch fries	1	640	51	6	45	11	44
Grilled chicken club sandwich	1	450	33	3	30	40	17
Grilled chicken sandwich	1	370	40	3	37	31	9
Half pound double Champ	1	740	30	3	27	39	52
Half pound double Champ w/ cheese	1	790	34	4	30	42	54
Homestyle chicken strip sandwich	1	670	50	4	46	27	41
Homestyle chicken strips meal	2 pc	670	58	5	53	27	37
Homestyle chicken strips meal	3 pc	890	77	7	70	36	49
Philly cheesesteak burger	1	500	38	3	35	29	26
Quarter pound bacon cheese Champ	1	630	35	5	30	29	41
Quarter pound Champ	1	490	32	4	28	22	30
Quarter pound Champ w/ cheese	1	580	33	4	29	24	39
Rallyburger	1	390	32	3	29	16	22

	SERVING SIZE	CALORIES	TOTAL CARBS (g)	FIBER (g)	NET CARBS (g)	PROTEIN (g)	FAT (g)
Checkers (cont.)	...	...	.	.	.	.	.
Rallyburger w/ cheese	1	420	33	3	30	18	24
Screamin' chicken strip sandwich	1	650	45	3	42	25	41
Screamin' chicken strips meal	2 pc	670	59	6	53	23	38
Screamin' chicken strips meal	3 pc	970	82	8	74	36	55
Spicy chicken sandwich	1	550	39	3	36	17	37
Strawberry shake, medium	1	440	71	0	71	9	13
Triple cheeseburger	1	690	33	4	29	43	43
Vanilla shake, medium	1	410	64	0	64	10	13
Chinese Restaurant – see	...	...	.	.	.	.	.
Panda Express Chinese Food	...	...	.	.	.	.	.
Chipotle Mexican Grill	...	...	.	.	.	.	.
Barbacoa	4 oz	170	2	0	2	24	7
Black beans	4 oz	120	23	11	12	7	1
Carnitas	4 oz	190	1	0	1	27	8
Cheese	1 oz	100	0	0	0	8	9
Chicken	4 oz	190	1	0	1	32	7
Chips	4 oz	570	73	8	65	8	27
Cilantro-lime rice	3 oz	130	23	0	23	2	3
Corn salsa	3.5 oz	80	15	3	12	3	2
Crispy taco shell	1	60	9	1	8	Tr	2
Fajita vegetables	2.5 oz	20	4	1	3	1	Tr
Flour tortilla, burrito	1	290	44	2	42	7	9

	SERVING SIZE	CALORIES	TOTAL CARBS (g)	FIBER (g)	NET CARBS (g)	PROTEIN (g)	FAT (g)
Chipotle Mexican Grill (cont.)	...	...	.	.	.	.	.
Flour tortilla, taco	1	90	13	Tr	13	2	3
Green tomatillo salsa	2 fl oz	15	3	1	2	1	0
Guacamole	3.5 oz	150	8	6	2	2	13
Pinto beans	4 oz	120	22	10	12	7	1
Red tomatillo salsa	2 fl oz	40	8	4	4	2	1
Romaine lettuce, salad	2.5 oz	10	2	1	1	1	0
Romaine lettuce, taco	1 oz	5	1	1	0	0	0
Sour cream	2 oz	120	2	0	2	2	10
Steak	4 oz	190	2	0	2	30	7
Tomato salsa	3.5 oz	20	4	Tr	4	1	0
Vinaigrette	2 fl oz	260	12	1	11	0	25
Church's Chicken	...	...	.	.	.	.	.
Apple pie	1	260	39	1	38	2	11
BBQ sauce	1 pkg	30	7	0	7	0	0
Bigger better chicken sandwich w/ cheese	1	510	46	4	42	20	27
Cajun rice	1 svg	130	16	Tr	16	1	7
Cole slaw	1 svg	150	15	2	13	1	10
Collard greens	1 svg	25	5	2	3	2	0
Corn on the cob	1 svg	140	24	9	15	4	3
Country fried steak sandwich	1	490	38	2	36	13	32
Country fried steak w/ white gravy	2 pc	610	31	2	29	24	43
Country fried steak w/ white gravy	1 pc	470	36	1	35	21	28
Creamy jalapeno sauce	1 pkg	100	1	0	1	0	11

	SERVING SIZE	CALORIES	TOTAL CARBS (g)	FIBER (g)	NET CARBS (g)	PROTEIN (g)	FAT (g)
Church's Chicken	...	...	.	.	.	.	.
(cont.)							
Crunchy tenders	1 pc	120	6	Tr	6	12	6
Edward's double lemon pie	1	300	39	0	39	5	14
Edward's strawberry cream cheese pie	1	280	32	2	30	4	15
French fries	1 svg	290	38	4	34	3	14
Honey	1 pkg	25	7	0	7	0	0
Honey butter biscuits	1	240	28	1	27	3	12
Honey mustard sauce	1 pkg	110	4	0	4	0	11
Hot sauce	1 pkg	20	0	0	0	0	0
Jalapeno bombers	4 pc	240	29	3	26	8	10
Ketchup	1 pkg	20	5	0	5	0	0
Macaroni & cheese	1 svg	210	23	1	22	8	11
Mashed potatoes & gravy	1 svg	70	12	1	11	2	2
Okra	1 svg	350	36	5	31	3	22
Original breast	1	200	3	1	2	22	11
Original leg	1	110	3	0	3	10	6
Original thigh	1	330	8	1	7	21	23
Original wing	1	300	7	3	4	27	19
Purple pepper sauce	1 pkg	45	12	0	12	0	0
Ranch sauce	1 pkg	130	1	0	1	0	13
Spicy breast	1	320	12	2	10	21	20
Spicy crunchy tenders	1 pc	140	7	4	3	11	7
Spicy fish fillet	1 pc	160	13	1	12	7	9
Spicy fish sandwich	1	320	25	2	23	10	20
Spicy leg	1	180	8	1	7	12	11

	SERVING SIZE	CALORIES	TOTAL CARBS (g)	FIBER (g)	NET CARBS (g)	PROTEIN (g)	FAT (g)
Church's Chicken	…	…	.	.	.	.	.
(cont.)							
Spicy thigh	1	480	20	2	18	22	35
Spicy wing	1	430	17	2	15	29	27
Sweet & sour sauce	1 pkg	30	8	0	8	0	0
Sweet corn nuggets	1 svg	600	72	5	67	7	29
Whole jalapeno peppers	2	10	2	1	1	0	0
Dairy Queen	…	…	.	.	.	.	.
(all listings medium size, unless noted)							
All-beef cheese dog	1	290	19	1	18	12	19
All-beef chili cheese dog	1	430	39	2	37	18	22
All-beef chili cheese foot-long dog	1	840	52	2	50	37	54
All-beef chili dog	1	290	24	1	23	11	17
All-beef foot-long hot dog	1	560	39	2	37	20	35
All-beef hot dog	1	250	21	1	20	9	14
Banana Cream Pie Blizzard	1	780	115	1	114	14	30
Banana malt	1	740	120	2	118	21	20
Banana shake	1	620	96	2	94	19	19
Banana split	1	520	94	3	91	9	13
Banana Split Blizzard	1	570	93	1	92	13	16
Banana sundae	1	330	53	1	52	8	10
Buster bar	1	480	45	2	43	11	31
Butterfinger blizzard	1	740	114	0	114	16	26

	SERVING SIZE	CALORIES	TOTAL CARBS (g)	FIBER (g)	NET CARBS (g)	PROTEIN (g)	FAT (g)
Dairy Queen (cont.)	...	...	.	.	.	.	.
Butterscotch dilly bar	1	210	24	0	24	3	11
Butterscotch dipped cone	1	490	59	0	59	9	23
Cappuccino *Heath* Blizzard	1	870	122	1	121	15	38
Caramel malt	1	960	163	0	163	22	24
Caramel shake	1	850	140	0	140	20	23
Caramel sundae	1	430	75	0	75	9	11
Cherry *Cheesequake* Blizzard	1	690	92	0	92	15	28
Cherry dilly bar	1	210	24	0	24	3	12
Cherry dipped cone	1	480	59	0	59	9	24
Cherry malt	1	800	130	0	130	20	22
Cherry shake	1	690	106	0	106	18	21
Cherry *Starkiss* bar	1	80	21	0	21	0	0
Cherry sundae	1	350	58	0	58	8	10
Chicken strip basket w/ country gravy	4 pc	1360	103	8	95	39	63
Chicken strip basket w/ country gravy	6 pc	1640	121	10	111	54	74
Choco Cherry Love Blizzard	1	730	94	1	93	14	33
Chocolate Chip Blizzard	1	880	96	2	94	14	50
Chocolate coated waffle cone w/ soft serve	1	540	77	1	76	10	21
Chocolate cone	1	340	54	0	54	9	10

	SERVING SIZE	CALORIES	TOTAL CARBS (g)	FIBER (g)	NET CARBS (g)	PROTEIN (g)	FAT (g)
Dairy Queen (cont.)	. . .	. . .	.	.	.	.	.
Chocolate covered strawberry waffle bowl sundae	1	790	99	2	97	10	40
Chocolate dilly bar	1	240	24	1	23	4	15
Chocolate dilly bar, mint	1	240	24	1	23	4	15
Chocolate dipped cone	1	470	60	1	59	9	22
Chocolate Extreme Blizzard	1	980	130	3	127	17	44
Chocolate malt	1	900	154	0	154	20	22
Chocolate shake	1	790	130	0	130	18	21
Chocolate sundae	1	400	70	0	70	8	10
Classic Grillburger	1	470	42	2	40	24	21
Cookie Dough Blizzard	1	1010	148	1	147	18	40
Crispy chicken salad	1	460	31	6	25	29	19
Crispy chicken sandwich	1	560	48	3	45	20	28
Crispy chicken sandwich w/ cheese	1	610	48	3	45	22	32
Crispy chicken wrap	1	290	17	2	15	11	16
Crispy Flame Thrower chicken sandwich	1	860	51	3	48	30	55
Crispy Flame Thrower chicken wrap	1	310	17	2	15	11	19
Dilly bar, no sugar added	1	190	24	5	19	3	13

	SERVING SIZE	CALORIES	TOTAL CARBS (g)	FIBER (g)	NET CARBS (g)	PROTEIN (g)	FAT (g)
Dairy Queen (cont.)	. . .	. . .	.	.	.	.	.
DQ frozen heart cake	1 piece	290	42	1	41	6	11
DQ frozen log cake	1 piece	310	44	1	43	6	12
DQ frozen round cake, 10″	1 piece	500	72	1	71	11	19
DQ frozen round cake, 8″	1 piece	410	59	1	58	9	15
DQ frozen sheet cake	1 piece	320	47	1	46	6	12
DQ fudge bar, no sugar added	1	50	13	6	7	4	0
DQ sandwich	1	190	31	1	30	4	5
DQ vanilla orange bar, no sugar added	1	60	18	6	12	2	0
Fab fudge waffle bowl sundae	1	750	108	1	107	10	30
French fries, large	1	500	70	5	65	6	21
French fries, regular	1	310	43	3	40	2	13
French Silk Pie Blizzard	1	920	117	2	115	15	44
Fudge brownie temptation waffle bowl sundae	1	970	120	3	117	14	49
Georgia *Mud Fudge* Blizzard	1	1010	114	4	110	19	54
Grilled chicken salad	1	280	14	4	10	31	11
Grilled chicken sandwich	1	370	32	1	31	24	16
Grilled chicken wrap	1	200	9	1	8	12	12

	SERVING SIZE	CALORIES	TOTAL CARBS (g)	FIBER (g)	NET CARBS (g)	PROTEIN (g)	FAT (g)
Dairy Queen (cont.)	. . .	. . .	.	.	.	.	.
Grilled Flame Thrower chicken sandwich	1	590	34	1	33	34	36
Half pound classic Grillburger w/ cheese	1	910	42	2	40	52	54
Half pound Flame Thrower Grillburger	1	1060	41	2	39	54	75
Half pound Grillburger	1	720	42	2	40	42	40
Half pound Grillburger w/ cheese	1	870	42	2	40	51	51
Hawaiian Blizzard	1	600	92	3	89	13	21
Health dilly bar	1	220	25	0	25	3	13
Heath Blizzard	1	920	126	1	125	16	41
Hot fudge malt	1	979	146	0	146	22	31
Hot fudge shake	1	850	123	0	123	20	30
Hot fudge sundae	1	440	66	0	66	9	14
Iron Griilled classic club sandwich	1	580	43	2	41	32	29
Iron Grilled turkey sandwich	1	530	42	2	40	29	25
Iron Grilled chicken quesadilla basket	1	1070	117	5	112	34	50
Iron Grilled supreme BLT sandwich	1	590	42	2	40	26	33
Iron Grilled veggie quesadilla basket	1	1020	114	9	105	26	46
M&M's Chocolate Candy Blizzard	1	840	127	1	126	16	29

	SERVING SIZE	CALORIES	TOTAL CARBS (g)	FIBER (g)	NET CARBS (g)	PROTEIN (g)	FAT (g)
Dairy Queen (cont.)	...	...	.	.	.	.	.
Marshmallow malt	1	900	157	0	157	20	22
Marshmallow shake	1	780	133	0	133	18	21
Marshmallow sundae	1	410	72	0	72	8	10
Mint *Oreo* Blizzard	1	740	116	1	115	14	25
Mocha Chip Blizzard	1	810	107	3	104	15	37
Nut & fudge waffle bowl sundae	1	880	99	4	95	17	47
Onion rings	1 svg	360	47	2	45	6	16
Oreo brownie earthquake	1	760	117	2	115	11	27
Oreo CheeseQuake Blizzard	1	820	108	1	107	16	35
Oreo Cookies Blizzard	1	680	100	1	99	14	25
Original bacon double cheeseburger	1	730	35	1	34	41	41
Original cheeseburger	1	400	34	1	33	19	18
Original double cheeseburger	1	640	34	1	33	34	34
Original double hamburger	1	540	33	1	32	29	26
Original hamburger	1	350	33	1	32	17	14
Peanut Buster parfait	1	700	94	2	92	16	30
Peanut Butter *Butterfinger* Blizzard	1	1050	122	5	117	20	54
Pineapple malt	1	750	123	1	122	20	20
Pineapple shake	1	650	99	1	98	18	21

	SERVING SIZE	CALORIES	TOTAL CARBS (g)	FIBER (g)	NET CARBS (g)	PROTEIN (g)	FAT (g)
Dairy Queen (cont.)	. . .	. . .	.	.	.	.	.
Pineapple sundae	1	340	54	0	54	8	10
Popcorn shrimp basket	1	990	115	8	107	18	49
Quarter pound Bacon Cheddar Grillburger	1	650	41	2	39	36	35
Quarter pound classic Grillburger w/ cheese	1	560	42	2	40	30	28
Quarter pound Flame Thrower Grillburger	1	780	41	2	39	34	52
Reese's Peanut Butter Cups Blizzard	1	760	101	2	99	18	31
Side salad	1	45	11	3	8	2	0
Snicker's Blizzard	1	850	123	2	121	18	33
Stars & Stripes Starkiss bar	1	80	21	0	21	0	0
Strawberry CheeseQuake Blizzard	1	690	92	0	92	15	28
Strawberry malt	1	770	128	1	127	21	20
Strawberry shake	1	650	97	1	96	18	21
Strawberry sundae	1	350	56	0	56	8	10
Tropical Blizzard	1	750	87	5	82	15	40
Turtle Pecan Cluster Blizzard	1	1050	127	3	124	17	54
Turtle waffle bowl sundae	1	810	116	2	114	12	34
Vanilla cone	1	330	53	0	53	9	10
Waffle cone w/ soft serve	1	420	67	0	67	10	13

	SERVING SIZE	CALORIES	TOTAL CARBS (g)	FIBER (g)	NET CARBS (g)	PROTEIN (g)	FAT (g)
Denny's	...	...	.	.	.	.	.
All-american slam	1	820	5	1	4	42	69
Appetizer sampler	1	1380	139	6	133	53	71
Apple crisp a la mode	1	750	134	4	130	7	21
Apple pie	1	510	72	3	69	4	23
Applesauce	1 svg	60	15	1	14	0	0
Bacon cheddar burger	1	1100	55	6	49	61	72
Bacon strips	4	180	2	0	2	14	13
Bacon, lettuce & tomato sandwich	1	570	36	2	34	20	37
Bagel & cream cheese	1	430	48	2	46	11	12
Baja salad w/ chicken	1	330	14	4	10	35	16
Baja salad w/ shrimp	1	280	12	3	9	21	17
Banana	1	110	29	4	25	1	0
Belgian waffle platter	1	650	31	2	29	20	50
Biscuit	1	210	25	0	25	3	11
Biscuits & sausage gravy	1	580	57	0	57	9	34
Black & bleu salad	1	270	6	1	5	24	16
Boca burger	1	500	62	10	52	30	15
Breaded chicken sandwich w/ honey mustard dressing	1	1190	104	5	99	44	65
Breaded shrimp	6 pc	190	20	2	18	9	8
Broccoli & cheddar soup	1	370	16	4	12	10	29
Butter roll	2 pc	260	38	1	37	5	9

	SERVING SIZE	CALORIES	TOTAL CARBS (g)	FIBER (g)	NET CARBS (g)	PROTEIN (g)	FAT (g)
Denny's (cont.)	...	...	.	.	.	.	.
Buttermilk pancakes, 3 each	1	510	102	3	99	12	6
Cheesecake	1	640	58	0	58	9	41
Cheesecake, no sugar added	1	290	23	0	23	6	23
Cheesy three pack appetizer	1	1940	164	8	156	52	125
Chicken deluxe salad, chicken strip	1	590	44	4	40	42	29
Chicken noodle soup	1	170	19	1	18	12	4
Chicken ranch melt	1	920	79	4	75	53	42
Chicken sausage patty	1	110	0	0	0	7	9
Chicken strips dinner	1	560	41	0	41	45	24
Chicken strips w/ buffalo sauce	1	730	53	1	52	57	32
Chicken wings w/ buffalo sauce	1	300	5	2	3	20	21
Cinnamon apples	1 svg	90	20	1	19	0	0
Clam chowder	1	270	24	2	22	5	17
Classic cheeseburger	1	930	56	5	51	49	58
Classic cheeseburger w/o cheese	1	770	56	5	51	39	45
Club sandwich	1	660	55	4	51	29	34
Coconut cream pie	1	630	65	1	64	6	39
Coleslaw	1 svg	260	15	3	12	2	22
Corn	1 svg	130	26	1	25	4	3
Cottage cheese	1 svg	70	5	0	5	9	2

	SERVING SIZE	CALORIES	TOTAL CARBS (g)	FIBER (g)	NET CARBS (g)	PROTEIN (g)	FAT (g)
Denny's (cont.)	...	...	.	.	.	.	.
Country fried potatoes	1 svg	390	30	10	20	3	28
Country fried steak w/ gravy	1	1000	54	6	48	51	65
Country-fried potatoes	1 svg	550	48	10	38	6	37
Country-fried steak & eggs	1	660	29	3	26	39	42
Cranberry pecan salad w/ chicken	1	250	11	1	10	32	8
Cranberry pecan salad w/ shrimp	1	190	9	1	8	18	9
Dippable veggies w/ ranch dressing	1	280	11	1	10	2	25
Double cheeseburger	1	1540	33	5	28	92	116
Egg whites	4 oz	50	1	0	1	11	0
Eggs, each	1	120	0	0	0	6	10
English muffin w/ margarine	1	180	25	1	24	4	3
Fabulous french toast platter	1	1010	93	5	88	43	52
Fit-fare boca burger	1	410	60	17	43	25	8
Fit-fare chicken sandwich w/ fruit	1	490	67	5	62	38	7
Fit-fare grilled chicken w/ vegetables & tomatoes	1	380	12	2	10	57	10
Fit-fare grilled tilapia	1	600	66	3	63	58	11
Fit-fare grilled chicken breast salad	1	290	15	4	11	36	10

	SERVING SIZE	CALORIES	TOTAL CARBS (g)	FIBER (g)	NET CARBS (g)	PROTEIN (g)	FAT (g)
Denny's (cont.)	. . .	. . .	.	.	.	.	.
French fries	1 svg	450	57	6	51	6	23
French silk pie	1	770	59	2	57	6	57
French toast slam	1	940	68	4	64	47	53
Fried shrimp w/ buffalo sauce	1	380	37	4	33	17	17
Garden salad w/o dressing	1	110	7	2	5	7	7
Garlic dinner bread	2 pc	170	21	1	20	4	9
Grand slam burrito	1	1160	106	6	100	43	62
Grand slamwich	1	1030	68	3	65	37	66
Granola w/ 8 oz milk	1	690	131	9	122	20	12
Grapes	1	55	29	4	25	1	0
Green beans, canned	1 svg	45	7	3	4	2	1
Green beans, frozen	1 svg	45	4	2	2	1	2
Grilled chicken	1	290	15	4	11	36	10
Grilled chicken dinner	1	280	4	0	4	55	4
Grilled chicken sandwich w/ honey mustard dressing	1	970	69	4	65	39	58
Grilled chicken sizzlin' skillet dinner	1	770	72	5	67	41	34
Grilled honey ham slice	1	110	1	0	1	14	5
Grilled shrimp skewer	1	90	0	0	0	14	4
Grilled shrimp skewers	1	370	39	2	37	32	10
Grits	1 svg	260	47	1	46	5	5

	SERVING SIZE	CALORIES	TOTAL CARBS (g)	FIBER (g)	NET CARBS (g)	PROTEIN (g)	FAT (g)
Denny's (cont.)	...	...	.	.	.	.	.
Half moons over my hammy	1	390	25	1	24	23	21
Ham & cheddar omelette	1	590	4	0	4	40	44
Hash browns	1 svg	210	26	2	24	2	12
Hash browns w/ cheese	1 svg	310	26	2	24	8	19
Hash browns w/ onions, cheese & gravy	1 svg	480	60	2	58	10	22
Heartland scramble	1	1150	97	7	90	40	66
Hershey's chocolate cake	1	580	75	2	73	6	28
Homestyle meatloaf w/ gravy	1	600	14	0	14	33	46
Hot fudge brownie a la mode	1	830	122	4	118	9	37
Lemon pepper tilapia	1	640	41	2	39	55	27
Lumberjack slam	1	850	60	3	57	45	46
Mashed potatoes	1 svg	170	76	1	75	2	7
Meat lover's scramble	1	1130	80	6	74	51	66
Milkshake, chocolate or vanilla	12 fl oz	560	76	Tr	76	11	26
Moons over my hammy	1	780	50	2	48	46	42
Mozzarella cheese sticks	1 svg	750	195	1	194	16	40
Mushroom swiss burger	1	900	59	6	53	47	54

	SERVING SIZE	CALORIES	TOTAL CARBS (g)	FIBER (g)	NET CARBS (g)	PROTEIN (g)	FAT (g)
Denny's (cont.)	. . .	. . .	.	.	.	.	.
Mushroom swiss chopped steak	1	930	18	1	17	46	75
Oatmeal w/ 8 oz milk	1	270	37	4	33	14	7
Onion rings	1 svg	520	48	3	45	6	36
Pancake puppies, 6 each	1	390	67	2	65	6	12
Pancakes, 3 each	1	510	102	3	99	12	6
Prime rib sizzlin' breakfast skillet	1	850	77	6	71	41	40
Prime rib sizzlin' skillet dinner	1	900	77	5	72	49	42
Sausage links	4	370	4	3	1	9	34
Seasonal fruit	1 svg	70	18	3	15	1	0
Seasoned fries	1 svg	510	48	5	43	6	33
Slamburger	1	750	13	2	11	41	60
Smokin' Q three pack appetizer	1	1870	179	9	170	62	106
Smothered cheese fries	1 svg	870	75	7	68	27	52
Southwestern sizzlin skillet	1	990	71	6	65	35	61
Spicy buffalo chicken melt	1	940	81	4	77	46	46
Super bird sandwich	1	560	43	2	41	38	27
Super grand slamwich	1	1320	71	4	67	53	89
Sweet & tangy BBQ chicken strips	1	820	83	2	81	58	30
Sweet & tangy BBQ chicken wings	1	420	41	1	40	21	19

	SERVING SIZE	CALORIES	TOTAL CARBS (g)	FIBER (g)	NET CARBS (g)	PROTEIN (g)	FAT (g)
Denny's (cont.)	...	...	.	.	.	.	.
Sweet & tangy BBQ shrimp	1	460	66	4	62	18	14
T-bone steak	1	740	0	0	0	59	56
T-bone steak & breaded shrimp	1	920	20	2	18	68	64
T-bone steak & eggs	1	780	4	0	4	110	36
T-bone steak & shrimp skewer	1	830	0	0	0	72	60
Toast w/ margarine	1 slice	130	16	1	15	3	7
Tomato slices	3	10	2	1	1	1	0
Top sirloin steak	1	220	1	0	1	41	6
Top sirloin steak & breaded shrimp	1	440	23	2	21	52	15
Top sirloin steak & eggs	1	420	1	0	1	54	21
Top sirloin steak & shrimp skewers	1	310	1	0	1	55	9
Turkey bacon	2 pc	80	0	0	0	8	4
Two egg breakfast	1	200	1	0	1	13	15
Ultimate omelette	1	670	8	2	6	36	54
Vegetable beef soup	1	120	18	3	15	10	1
Vegetable rice pilaf	1 svg	200	37	1	36	4	3
Veggie-cheese omelette	1	500	10	2	8	29	37
Western burger	1	1300	83	6	77	58	82
Wheat pancakes, 2 each	1	310	64	8	56	10	2
Yogurt, lowfat	6 oz	160	30	0	30	6	2
Zesty nachos	1	1150	138	11	127	46	49

	SERVING SIZE	CALORIES	TOTAL CARBS (g)	FIBER (g)	NET CARBS (g)	PROTEIN (g)	FAT (g)
Domino's Pizza	. . .	. . .	.	.	.	.	.
Crusts, plain (⅛ of 12" pizza)	. . .	. . .	.	.	.	.	.
Hand tossed	1 slice	120	22	1	21	4	2
Thin crust	1 slice	80	12	1	11	2	4
Deep dish	1 slice	160	24	3	21	4	5
Feast pizza toppings (⅛ of 12" pizza)	. . .	. . .	.	.	.	.	.
America's favorite	1 slice	120	4	1	3	6	10
Bacon cheeseburger	1 slice	140	3	1	2	8	11
Barbecue	1 slice	130	8	0	8	7	8
Deluxe	1 slice	100	4	1	3	5	8
Extravaganzza	1 slice	150	5	1	4	9	12
Hawaiian	1 slice	90	5	1	4	6	6
Meatzza	1 slice	150	4	1	3	9	11
Pepperoni	1 slice	130	4	1	3	7	11
Philly Cheese Steak	1 slice	100	1	0	1	7	7
Vegi	1 slice	80	4	1	3	5	6
Side Orders & Condiments	. . .	. . .	.	.	.	.	.
Barbeque buffalo wings	2 pc	230	6	0	6	17	14
Blue cheese dipping sauce	1 svg	210	2	0	2	1	22
Blue cheese dressing	1 pkg	230	2	0	2	2	24
Breadsticks	1 pc	110	11	0	11	2	6
Buffalo chicken kickers	2 pc	100	7	1	6	9	5
Buttermilk ranch dressing	1 pkg	220	2	0	2	1	24

	SERVING SIZE	CALORIES	TOTAL CARBS (g)	FIBER (g)	NET CARBS (g)	PROTEIN (g)	FAT (g)
Domino's Pizza	...	...	.	.	.	.	.
(cont.)							
Cheesy bread	1 pc	120	11	0	11	4	6
Cinna Stix	1 pc	120	14	1	13	2	6
Creamy caesar dressing	1 pkg	210	2	0	2	1	22
Croutons	1 pkg	45	6	0	6	1	2
Garden fresh salad w/o dressing	1 svg	70	5	2	3	4	4
Garlic dipping sauce	1 svg	250	0	0	0	0	28
Golden Italian dressing	1 pkg	220	2	0	2	0	23
Grilled chicken Caesar salad w/o dressing	1 svg	100	6	2	4	10	5
Hot buffalo wings	2 pc	200	2	0	2	16	14
Hot dipping sauce	1 svg	50	3	0	3	0	5
Italian dipping sauce	1 svg	25	5	1	4	1	0
Light Italian dressing	1 pkg	20	2	0	2	0	1
Marinara dipping sauce	1 svg	25	5	1	4	1	0
Parmesan peppercorn dipping sauce	1 svg	190	2	0	2	0	21
Ranch dipping sauce	1 svg	190	2	0	2	0	21
Sweet icing	1 svg	250	57	0	57	0	3
Dunkin' Donuts	...	...	.	.	.	.	.
Bagels	...	...	...	...	.	.	.
Cinnamon raisin	1	370	72	3	69	13	4

	SERVING SIZE	CALORIES	TOTAL CARBS (g)	FIBER (g)	NET CARBS (g)	PROTEIN (g)	FAT (g)
Dunkin' Donuts (cont.)	. . .	. . .	.	.	.	.	.
Everything	1	360	74	3	71	15	5
Garlic	1	350	76	4	72	15	4
Onion	1	340	65	3	62	12	4
Plain	1	330	71	3	68	14	3
Poppyseed	1	370	73	3	70	15	6
Salt	1	330	71	3	68	14	3
Sesame	1	370	72	3	69	16	7
Multigrain	1	400	65	10	55	18	9
Wheat	1	350	66	5	61	13	4
Cream cheese	. . .	. . .	. . .	.	.	.	.
Plain	1 pkt	150	3	0	3	3	15
Reduced fat	1 pkt	100	5	0	5	4	8
Reduced fat smoked salmon	1 pkt	140	6	0	6	4	11
Reduced fat blueberry	1 pkt	150	15	0	15	2	9
Reduced fat strawberry	1 pkt	150	15	0	15	2	10
Reduced fat veggie	1 pkt	120	6	0	6	2	10
Reduced fat onion & chive	1 pkt	130	6	0	6	3	11
Cookies	. . .	. . .	. . .	.	.	.	.
Chocolate chunk	1	540	80	3	77	7	23
Oatmeal raisin	1	480	83	5	78	8	14
Danish	. . .	. . .	. . .	.	.	.	.
Apple cheese	1	330	41	1	40	4	16
Cheese	1	330	39	1	38	5	17
Strawberry cheese	1	320	40	1	39	4	16
Donuts	. . .	. . .	. . .	.	.	.	.
Apple crumb	1	460	80	2	78	4	14

	SERVING SIZE	CALORIES	TOTAL CARBS (g)	FIBER (g)	NET CARBS (g)	PROTEIN (g)	FAT (g)
Dunkin' Donuts (cont.)	...	...	.	.	.	.	.
Apple & spice	1	240	32	1	31	3	11
Bavarian kreme	1	250	31	1	30	3	12
Black raspberry	1	210	32	1	31	3	8
Blueberry cake	1	330	38	1	37	3	18
Blueberry crumb	1	470	84	2	82	4	14
Boston kreme	1	280	38	1	37	3	12
Chocolate coconut cake	1	400	49	2	47	3	22
Chocolate frosted cake	1	340	38	1	37	3	19
Chocolate frosted	1	230	32	1	31	3	10
Chocolate glazed cake	1	280	33	1	32	3	15
Chocolate kreme filled	1	310	37	1	36	4	16
Cinnamon cake	1	290	30	1	29	3	18
Double chocolate cake	1	290	34	1	33	3	16
French cruller	1	250	18	0	18	2	20
Glazed cake	1	320	37	1	36	3	18
Glazed	1	220	31	1	30	3	9
Jelly filled	1	260	36	1	35	3	11
Maple frosted	1	230	33	1	32	3	10
Marble frosted	1	230	32	1	31	3	10
Old fashioned cake	1	280	27	1	26	3	18
Powdered cake	1	300	30	1	29	3	18
Strawberry	1	210	32	1	31	3	8
Strawberry frosted	1	230	33	1	32	3	10
Sugar raised	1	190	22	1	21	3	9
Vanilla kreme filled	1	320	37	1	36	3	17

	SERVING SIZE	CALORIES	TOTAL CARBS (g)	FIBER (g)	NET CARBS (g)	PROTEIN (g)	FAT (g)
Dunkin' Donuts (cont.)	...	...	.	.	.	.	.
Whole white glazed cake	1	310	32	1	31	4	19
Donut–Fancies	...	...	.	.	.	.	.
Apple fritter	1	400	63	2	61	5	15
Bow tie donut	1	310	39	1	38	4	15
Chocolate frosted coffee roll	1	380	50	2	48	5	19
Chocolate iced Bismarck	1	350	53	1	52	4	14
Coffee roll	1	370	49	2	47	5	18
Éclair	1	350	53	1	52	4	14
Glazed fritter	1	400	63	2	61	5	15
Maple frosted coffee roll	1	380	50	2	48	5	18
Vanilla frosted coffee roll	1	380	50	2	48	5	18
Donut–Munchkins	...	...	.	.	.	.	.
Cinnamon cake	1	60	6	0	6	1	3
Glazed	1	50	7	0	7	1	3
Glazed cake	1	60	8	0	8	1	3
Glazed chocolate cake	1	60	8	0	8	1	3
Jelly filled	1	60	8	0	8	1	3
Plain cake	1	50	5	0	5	1	3
Powdered cake	1	60	6	0	6	1	4
Sugar raised	1	40	5	0	5	1	3
Donut–Sticks	...	...	.	.	.	.	.
Cinnamon cake	1	310	30	1	29	3	20
Glazed cake	1	340	38	1	37	3	20
Glazed chocolate cake	1	390	40	2	38	3	25
Jelly	1	400	54	1	53	3	20
Plain cake	1	300	26	1	25	3	20

	SERVING SIZE	CALORIES	TOTAL CARBS (g)	FIBER (g)	NET CARBS (g)	PROTEIN (g)	FAT (g)
Dunkin' Donuts (cont.)	...	...	.	.	.	.	.
Powdered cake	1	320	31	1	30	3	20
Muffins	...	...	.	.	.	.	.
Blueberry	1	510	87	3	84	6	16
Chocolate chip	1	630	98	5	93	8	23
Coffee cake	1	620	93	2	91	7	25
Corn	1	510	84	2	82	6	17
Honey bran raisin	1	500	86	9	77	7	14
Reduced fat blueberry	1	450	86	3	83	6	10
Other Misc. Items	...	...	...	.	.	.	.
Biscuit, plain	1	280	32	1	31	5	14
Brownie	1	430	56	1	55	3	23
Cinnamon twist	1	210	25	1	24	3	11
Croissant, plain	1	310	35	1	34	7	16
English muffin	1	160	31	2	29	6	2
Sandwiches, Breakfast type	...	...	.	.	.	.	.
Bagel w/ egg, bacon, cheese	1	530	76	3	73	26	18
Bagel w/ egg, ham, cheese	1	520	75	3	72	28	17
Bagel w/ egg, sausage, cheese	1	660	76	3	73	30	29
Biscuit w/ egg & cheese	1	430	36	1	35	13	26
Biscuit w/ sausage, egg, cheese	1	600	37	1	36	20	40
Croissant w/ egg, ham, cheese	1	510	39	1	38	21	30
English muffin w/egg, cheese	1	320	34	2	32	14	13

	SERVING SIZE	CALORIES	TOTAL CARBS (g)	FIBER (g)	NET CARBS (g)	PROTEIN (g)	FAT (g)
Dunkin' Donuts (cont.)	...	...	.	.	.	.	.
English muffin w/ egg, bacon & cheese	...	...	.	.	.	.	.
	1	360	35	2	33	18	16
English muffin w/ egg, ham, & cheese	...	...	.	.	.	.	.
	1	350	35	2	33	21	15
Beverages	...	...	.	.	.	.	.
Cappuccino	10 oz	80	7	0	7	4	4
Cappuccino with sugar	10 oz	140	24	0	24	4	4
Coffee	10 oz	5	1	0	1	0	0
Coffee with cream	10 oz	60	2	0	2	1	6
Coffee with cream and sugar	10 oz	120	19	0	19	1	6
Coffee with milk	10 oz	25	2	0	2	1	1
Coffee with milk and sugar	10 oz	80	20	0	20	1	1
Coffee with skim milk	10 oz	15	3	0	3	2	0
Coffee w/ skim milk and sugar	10 oz	70	20	0	20	2	0
Coffee with sugar	10 oz	60	18	0	18	0	0
Coffee coolatta with cream	16 oz	330	28	0	28	3	23
Coffee coolatta with milk	16 oz	170	29	0	29	4	4
Coffee coolatta with skim milk	16 oz	140	30	0	30	4	0
Coolatta, grape	16 oz	240	59	0	59	0	0
Coolatta, orange mango	16 oz	220	52	0	52	1	0
Coolatta, strawberry fruit	16 oz	300	72	0	72	0	0

	SERVING SIZE	CALORIES	TOTAL CARBS (g)	FIBER (g)	NET CARBS (g)	PROTEIN (g)	FAT (g)
Dunkin' Donuts (cont.)	. . .	. . .	.	.	.	.	.
Coolatta, vanilla bean	16 oz	430	90	0	90	3	6
Coolatta, watermelon	16 oz	250	60	0	60	0	0
Dunkaccino	10 oz	230	35	1	34	2	11
Espresso	1.75 oz	0	0	0	0	0	0
Espresso with sugar	1.75 oz	30	7	0	7	0	0
Hot chocolate	10 oz	210	39	2	37	2	7
Latte, plain	10 oz	120	10	0	10	6	6
Latte with sugar	10 oz	170	27	0	27	6	6
Latte w/ Caramel swirl	10 oz	220	35	0	35	8	6
Latte w/ Mocha swirl	10 oz	220	35	1	34	7	6
Iced coffee	16 oz	10	2	0	2	1	0
Iced coffee with cream	16 oz	70	3	0	3	1	6
Iced coffee w/ cream and sugar	16 oz	120	20	0	20	1	6
Iced coffee with milk	16 oz	30	3	0	3	2	1
Iced coffee w/ milk and sugar	16 oz	90	21	0	21	2	1
Iced coffee with skim milk	16 oz	20	3	0	3	2	0
Iced coffee w/ skim milk, sugar	16 oz	80	21	0	21	2	0
Iced coffee with sugar	16 oz	70	19	0	19	1	0
Iced latte	16 oz	120	10	0	10	6	6
Iced latte with sugar	16 oz	170	27	0	27	6	6

	SERVING SIZE	CALORIES	TOTAL CARBS (g)	FIBER (g)	NET CARBS (g)	PROTEIN (g)	FAT (g)
Dunkin' Donuts (cont.)	. . .	. . .	.	.	.	.	.
Iced caramel swirl latte	16 oz	220	35	0	35	8	6
Iced mocha swirl latte	16 oz	220	35	1	34	7	6
Vanilla chai	14 oz	330	53	0	53	11	9
Tea, plain, w/o milk or sugar	. . .	. . .	.	.	.	.	.
Decaffeinated tea	10 oz	0	0	0	0	0	0
Earl Grey tea	10 oz	0	0	0	0	0	0
English breakfast tea	10 oz	0	0	0	0	0	0
Green tea	10 oz	0	0	0	0	0	0
Tea w/ regular milk, no sugar	10 oz	20	1	0	1	1	1
Tea w/ regular milk and sugar	10 oz	80	19	0	19	1	1
Tea w/ skim milk, no sugar	10 oz	10	2	0	2	1	0
Tea w/ skim milk and sugar	10 oz	70	19	0	19	1	0
Einstein Bros Bagels	. . .	. . .	.	.	.	.	.
Apple cream cheese bagel	1	550	89	4	85	11	17
Asiago cheese bagel	1	330	59	2	57	15	5
Asiago cheese bagel pretzel	1	300	52	2	50	11	7
Bacon & spinach panini	1	860	66	6	60	27	51
Bagel croutons	1 oz	100	15	1	14	2	4
Blueberry bagel	1	290	64	3	61	9	2
Blueberry muffin	1	480	65	2	63	6	22

	SERVING SIZE	CALORIES	TOTAL CARBS (g)	FIBER (g)	NET CARBS (g)	PROTEIN (g)	FAT (g)
Einstein Bros Bagels (cont.)	...	...	.	.	.	.	.
Blueberry reduced fat whipped cream cheese	2 Tbsp	70	6	0	6	1	5
Braided challah roll	1	220	41	1	40	8	4
Bros bistro salad	1	820	38	7	31	14	68
Bros bistro salad w/ chicken	1	940	39	7	32	36	71
Caesar dressing	2 Tbsp	150	1	0	1	1	16
Caesar salad	1	690	18	4	14	18	63
Caesar salad w/ chicken	1	820	20	4	16	42	66
California chicken wrap	1	630	63	8	55	33	28
Candied walnuts	1.5 oz	260	9	3	6	4	22
Cheese pizza bagel	1	420	63	3	60	23	12
Cheesy garlic & herb pizza bagel	1	500	65	2	63	24	19
Chicken chipotle salad	1	710	54	10	44	34	41
Chicken noodle soup	1 cup	120	14	1	13	5	4
Chile lime dressing	2 Tbsp	60	5	0	5	1	4
Chipotle salad	1	590	53	10	43	13	38
Chipotle turkey wrap	1	730	70	9	61	34	37
Chocolate chip bagel	1	290	60	3	57	10	3
Chocolate chip coffee cake	1	760	110	2	108	6	34
Chocolate mudslide cookie	1	320	46	1	45	4	17
Ciabatta bread	1	290	60	2	58	10	3

	SERVING SIZE	CALORIES	TOTAL CARBS (g)	FIBER (g)	NET CARBS (g)	PROTEIN (g)	FAT (g)
Einstein Bros	. . .	. . .	.	.	.	.	.
Bagels (cont.)							
Cinnamon raisin swirl bagel	1	290	64	3	61	10	1
Cinnamon stix	1	370	41	2	39	5	21
Cinnamon sugar bagel pretzel	1	320	66	3	63	8	5
Cinnamon sugar bagel, Chicago style	1	310	66	3	63	10	3
Cinnamon walnut strudel	1	630	56	4	52	9	42
Club mex sandwich, on challah	1	750	46	2	44	36	49
Cole slaw	1 svg	230	12	3	9	2	21
Corn crab chowder	1 cup	280	18	1	17	8	18
Cranberry bagel	1	290	64	3	61	9	1
Deli bacon sandwich	1	830	52	4	48	39	52
Deli chicken salad sandwich	1	460	47	4	43	28	18
Deli ham sandwich	1	520	48	4	44	26	26
Deli pastrami sandwich	1	630	53	5	48	34	33
Deli tuna salad sandwich	1	440	50	4	46	29	15
Deli turkey & swiss sandwich	1	690	49	4	45	36	41
Dutch apple bagel	1	340	66	2	64	8	7
Egg bagel	1	300	52	2	50	12	6
Egg way sandwich w/ bacon	1	580	59	2	57	33	24

	SERVING SIZE	CALORIES	TOTAL CARBS (g)	FIBER (g)	NET CARBS (g)	PROTEIN (g)	FAT (g)
Einstein Bros Bagels (cont.)	...	...	.	.	.	.	.
Egg way sandwich w/ black forest ham	1	570	62	2	60	37	21
Egg way sandwich w/ sausage	1	600	63	2	61	38	24
Egg way sandwich, original	1	530	62	2	60	30	20
Egg way sandwich, spinach, mushroom & swiss omelette	1	540	65	3	62	29	20
Elvis' favorite bagel	1	700	98	8	90	24	30
Everything bagel	1	270	56	2	54	10	2
Fruit and yogurt parfait	1	230	42	4	38	12	2
Fruit salad, side	1	140	36	3	33	2	0
Fudge brownie	1	510	74	2	72	6	25
Garden vegetable reduced fat whipped cream cheese	2 Tbsp	60	3	0	3	1	5
Garlic dip'd bagel	1	290	60	2	58	10	3
Garlic herb reduced fat whipped cream cheese	2 Tbsp	60	3	0	3	1	5
Good grains bagel	1	290	62	4	58	10	3
Green chile bagel	1	370	62	2	60	16	8
Grilled chicken, bacon & swiss sandwich	1	750	45	2	43	40	46
Ham deli melt	1	510	62	3	59	36	16
Heavenly chocolate chunk cookie	1	360	48	2	46	4	18

	SERVING SIZE	CALORIES	TOTAL CARBS (g)	FIBER (g)	NET CARBS (g)	PROTEIN (g)	FAT (g)
Einstein Bros Bagels (cont.)	...	...	.	.	.	.	.
Honey almond reduced fat whipped cream cheese	2 Tbsp	70	6	0	6	1	5
Honey whole wheat bagel	1	270	61	3	58	9	1
Iced sugar cookie	1	480	76	1	75	4	15
Italian chicken panini	1	800	66	5	61	35	40
Italian wedding	1 cup	160	15	2	13	11	6
Jalapeno salsa reduced fat whipped cream cheese	2 Tbsp	60	3	0	3	1	5
Kettle classic natural potato chips	1 oz	150	15	1	14	2	9
Lemon pound cake	1	440	69	1	68	7	16
Lox & bagels	1	520	66	3	63	25	21
Marshmallow crispy treat	1	220	48	0	48	3	4
Mini chocolate mudslide cookie	1	160	23	1	22	2	8
Mini heavenly chocolate chunk cookie	1	180	24	1	23	2	9
Mini iced sugar cookie	1	230	39	1	38	2	7
Mini oatmeal raisin cookie	1	160	27	1	26	2	5
Mixed berry coffee cake	1	710	110	2	108	5	29
Multigrain bread	1 slice	130	23	2	21	5	3

	SERVING SIZE	CALORIES	TOTAL CARBS (g)	FIBER (g)	NET CARBS (g)	PROTEIN (g)	FAT (g)
Einstein Bros	...	...	.	.	.	.	.
Bagels (cont.)							
Oatmeal raisin cookie	1	320	54	2	52	5	11
Onion & chive whipped cream cheese	2 Tbsp	70	3	0	3	1	6
Onion bagel	1	270	59	2	57	9	2
Onion dip'd bagel	1	270	59	2	57	9	1
Original asiago bagel dog	1	490	56	2	54	22	21
Original asiago bagel dog w/ cheddar cheese	1	560	56	2	54	26	27
Original bagel dog	1	470	56	2	54	20	20
Original bagel dog w/ cheddar cheese	1	550	56	2	54	25	26
Pastrami deli melt	1	540	64	3	61	38	17
Pepperoni pizza bagel	1	470	63	3	60	24	16
Plain bagel	1	260	56	2	54	9	1
Plain bagel pretzel	1	270	52	2	50	8	5
Plain reduced fat whipped cream cheese	2 Tbsp	60	2	0	2	1	5
Plain whipped cream cheese	2 Tbsp	70	1	0	1	1	7
Poppy dip'd bagel	1	280	56	2	54	10	3
Potato bagel	1	260	58	2	56	9	1
Power bagel, fruit & nut	1	380	72	5	67	13	6
Pumpernickel bagel	1	250	55	3	52	9	2
Rachel, overstuffed	1	1030	53	2	51	54	68

	SERVING SIZE	CALORIES	TOTAL CARBS (g)	FIBER (g)	NET CARBS (g)	PROTEIN (g)	FAT (g)
Einstein Bros Bagels (cont.)	...	...	.	.		.	.
Rachel, regular	1	910	51	2	49	36	64
Raspberry vinaigrette dressing	2 Tbsp	160	8	0	8	0	14
Reuben, overstuffed	1	760	49	3	46	51	42
Reuben, regular	1	650	47	3	44	34	38
Roasted turkey & swiss sandwich	1	690	49	4	45	35	41
Salt bagel pretzel	1	270	52	2	50	8	5
Santa Fe wrap	1	720	60	7	53	37	37
Sausage ranchero panini	1	680	64	4	60	32	29
Seafood minestrone	1 cup	130	16	2	14	8	5
Sesame dip'd bagel	1	280	56	2	54	10	3
Six-cheese bagel	1	350	60	2	58	16	6
Smoked salmon whipped cream cheese	2 Tbsp	60	2	0	2	1	6
Spicy Elmo wrap	1	720	56	6	50	34	41
Spinach & mushroom pizza bagel	1	580	70	4	66	26	25
Spinach florentine bagel	1	360	61	2	59	16	8
Strawberry cream cheese bagel	1	480	82	3	79	11	12
Strawberry reduced fat whipped cream cheese	2 Tbsp	70	5	0	5	1	5
Strawberry white chocolate muffin	1	550	78	1	77	7	25

	SERVING SIZE	CALORIES	TOTAL CARBS (g)	FIBER (g)	NET CARBS (g)	PROTEIN (g)	FAT (g)
Einstein Bros	...	...	.	.	.	.	.
Bagels (cont.)							
Sundried tomato bagel	1	270	58	3	55	10	2
Sundried tomato basil reduced fat whipped cream cheese	2 Tbsp	60	2	0	2	1	5
Tasty turkey sandwich, on asiago bagel	1	580	69	3	66	37	20
Traditional potato salad	1/2 cup	360	20	2	18	3	29
Tuna salad deli melt	1	590	64	3	61	38	23
Turkey chili	1 cup	220	24	5	19	20	7
Turkey club panini	1	790	66	6	60	34	41
Turkey deli melt	1	510	62	3	59	38	15
Turkey Rachel, overstuffed	1	1100	54	2	52	59	74
Turkey Rachel, regular	1	870	49	1	48	38	62
Turkey reuben, overstuffed	1	680	45	3	42	54	37
Turkey reuben, regular	1	610	45	3	42	36	36
Veg out sandwich, on sesame seed bagel	1	440	66	4	62	17	14
Vegetable breakfast panini	1	730	68	4	64	26	36
Vegetarian broccoli cheese	1 cup	290	16	2	14	14	20
Veggie deli melt	1	640	76	5	71	24	29

	SERVING SIZE	CALORIES	TOTAL CARBS (g)	FIBER (g)	NET CARBS (g)	PROTEIN (g)	FAT (g)
El Pollo Loco	. . .	. . .	.	.		.	.
Avocado salsa	1 svg	40	2	1	1	0	4
BBQ black beans	1 svg	200	36	4	32	7	3
BRC burrito	1	440	68	6	62	15	12
Caramel flan	1	260	34	0	34	5	12
Cheese quesadilla	1	420	35	2	33	19	23
Chicken Caesar Bowl	1	490	44	2	42	28	22
Chicken caesar salad, no dressing	1	230	18	3	15	25	7
Chicken soft taco	1	260	18	2	16	16	12
Chicken taquito w/ avocado salsa	1	230	20	2	18	10	12
Chicken tortilla soup, large	1	450	37	5	32	34	20
Chicken tortilla soup, regular	1	210	18	2	16	16	9
Chicken tortilla soup, regular, no tortilla strips	1	140	8	2	6	15	6
Chicken tortilla soup, small	1	160	14	2	12	10	8
Chicken tostada salad, no dressing	1	840	74	7	67	40	42
Chicken tostada salad, no dressing, no shell	1	410	39	5	34	33	13
Chips & guacamole	1 svg	250	26	4	22	3	14
Classic Chicken Burrito	1	550	69	6	63	31	17
Cole Slaw	1 svg	130	9	2	7	1	10
Corn cobbette	1	90	19	2	17	2	Tr

	SERVING SIZE	CALORIES	TOTAL CARBS (g)	FIBER (g)	NET CARBS (g)	PROTEIN (g)	FAT (g)
El Pollo Loco (cont.)	...	...	.	.	.	.	.
Corn tortilla, 6"	2	120	24	2	22	2	2
Creamy cilantro dressing, large	1 svg	440	3	0	3	3	46
Creamy cilantro dressing, light	1 pkt	70	6	0	6	1	5
Creamy cilantro dressing, regular	1 svg	190	1	0	1	1	20
Crunchy chicken taco	1	190	16	2	14	12	8
Flame-grilled chicken breast	1	220	0	0	0	36	9
Flame-grilled chicken breast, skinless	1	180	0	0	0	35	4
Flame-grilled chicken leg	1	90	0	0	0	12	4
Flame-grilled chicken thigh	1	220	0	0	0	21	15
Flame-grilled chicken wing	1	90	0	0	0	11	5
Flame-grilled chopped chicken breast meat	1	100	0	0	0	21	2
Flour tortilla, 6.5"	2	210	30	2	28	5	7
French fries	1 svg	330	42	4	38	4	17
Fresh vegetables w/ margarine	1 svg	60	8	3	5	2	3
Fresh vegetables w/o margarine	1 svg	35	8	3	5	2	0
Garden salad, small, no dressing	1	70	8	2	6	2	4

	SERVING SIZE	CALORIES	TOTAL CARBS (g)	FIBER (g)	NET CARBS (g)	PROTEIN (g)	FAT (g)
El Pollo Loco (cont.)	...	...	.	.	.	.	.
Garden salad, small, no dressing, no tortilla strips	1	35	4	1	3	2	2
Gravy	1 oz	10	2	0	2	0	0
Grilled chicken nachos	1	810	70	10	60	39	40
Grilled chicken tortilla roll, no sauce	1	390	37	3	34	26	16
Guacamole	1 svg	70	3	2	1	1	6
Horchata	20 oz	60	9	0	9	0	2
House salsa	1 svg	10	2	0	2	0	0
Jalapeno hot sauce	1 pkt	5	1	0	1	0	0
Ketchup	1 pkt	10	2	0	2	0	0
Light Italian dressing	1 pkt	20	2	0	2	0	1
Loco salad w/ creamy cilantro dressing	1	170	7	1	6	3	14
Macaroni & cheese	1 svg	280	28	0	28	11	17
Mashed potatoes	1 svg	110	23	2	21	2	2
Pico de gallo	1 svg	15	2	0	2	0	1
Pinto beans	1 svg	200	29	8	21	11	4
Queso sauce	1 svg	80	3	0	3	2	6
Ranch dressing	1 pkt	230	2	0	2	1	24
Refried beans w/ cheese	1 svg	270	36	10	26	14	7
Salsa de arbol	1 svg	10	2	0	2	0	0
Skinless breast meal	1	280	12	4	8	39	8
Sour cream	1 svg	80	1	0	1	1	7
Spanish rice	1 svg	220	45	1	44	4	2

	SERVING SIZE	CALORIES	TOTAL CARBS (g)	FIBER (g)	NET CARBS (g)	PROTEIN (g)	FAT (g)
El Pollo Loco (cont.)	...	...	.	.	.	.	.
Taco al carbon	1	150	17	1	16	11	5
The Original Pollo Bowl	1	690	106	12	94	40	10
Thousand island dressing	1 pkt	220	6	0	6	0	21
Tortilla chips	1 svg	170	23	2	21	2	8
Twice Grilled Burrito	1	840	56	6	50	66	39
Two churros	2	300	32	2	30	3	18
Ultimate grilled burrito	1	710	86	8	78	39	23
Ultimate Pollo Bowl	1	1050	110	13	97	71	34
Vanilla soft serve, cone, regular	1	320	53	0	53	8	8
Vanilla soft serve, cup	5 oz	300	48	0	48	8	8
Fatburger	...	...	.	.	.	.	.
American cheese, add-on	1	70	1	0	1	5	5
American cheese, Kingburger add-on	1	150	1	0	1	9	11
Baby Fat	1	400	37	2	35	17	21
Bacon & egg sandwich	1	350	37	1	36	18	16
Bacon, add-on	1	80	0	0	0	7	7
Big fat float	1	390	73	0	73	3	12
Cheddar cheese, add-on	1	110	1	0	1	7	9
Chili cheese fat fries	1 svg	590	53	6	47	21	33
Chili cheese hot dog	1	480	35	2	33	24	27

	SERVING SIZE	CALORIES	TOTAL CARBS (g)	FIBER (g)	NET CARBS (g)	PROTEIN (g)	FAT (g)
Fatburger (cont.)	...	...	.	.	.	.	.
Chili cheese skinny fries	1 svg	600	64	5	59	19	30
Chili cup	1	200	10	2	8	16	11
Chili cup w/ cheese & onions	1	320	12	2	10	23	20
Chili fat fries	1 svg	480	52	6	46	14	24
Chili skinny fries	1 svg	490	63	5	58	12	21
Chili, add-on	1	50	2	1	1	4	3
Chocolate shake	1	910	115	2	113	14	45
Cookies & ice cream shake	1	1180	163	2	161	18	59
Crispy chicken sandwich	1	560	53	2	51	26	27
Egg, add-on	1	90	0	0	0	6	7
Fat fries	1 svg	380	47	5	42	6	18
Fat salad wedge w/ chicken, no dressing	1	210	8	2	6	33	6
Fat salad wedge, no dressing	1	60	5	2	3	5	4
Fatburger	1	590	46	2	44	33	31
Fatburger, w/o bun	1	410	10	2	8	28	29
Fish sandwich	1	560	55	2	53	20	31
Grilled chicken sandwich	1	430	42	2	40	33	14
Grilled onions	1 svg	120	1	0	1	0	14
Hot dog	1	320	32	1	31	13	15
Kingburger	1	850	69	4	65	50	41
Lettuce	1 svg	5	1	0	1	0	0
Maui-banana shake	1	940	126	1	125	13	44
Mayonnaise	1 svg	90	1	0	1	0	10
Mustard	1 svg	5	0	0	0	0	0

	SERVING SIZE	CALORIES	TOTAL CARBS (g)	FIBER (g)	NET CARBS (g)	PROTEIN (g)	FAT (g)
Fatburger (cont.)	...	...	.	.	.	.	.
Onion rings	1 svg	540	64	4	60	7	29
Onions	1 svg	5	1	0	1	0	0
Peanut butter shake	1	950	114	1	113	14	53
Pickles	1 svg	5	1	0	1	0	0
Pickles, Kingburger	1 svg	5	1	0	1	0	0
Relish	1 svg	20	5	0	5	0	0
Sausage & egg sandwich	1	780	47	1	46	27	53
Skinny fries	1 svg	390	58	4	54	4	15
Spicy chicken sandwich	1	520	58	2	56	26	21
Strawberry shake	1	880	111	1	110	14	44
Tomato	1 svg	5	1	0	1	0	0
Tomato, Kingburger	1 svg	5	2	0	2	0	0
Turkeyburger	1	480	50	3	47	26	21
Vanilla shake	1	890	113	0	113	13	44
Veggieburger	1	510	60	11	49	33	20
Wing sauce	1 svg	50	6	0	6	0	4
Friendly's	...	...	.	.	.	.	.
All American burger	1	860	55	4	51	39	54
All American burger, side bacon	1	70	0	0	0	6	6
All American burger, side cheese	1	90	1	0	1	4	7
Apple juice, large	1	210	53	0	53	0	0
Apple juice, small	1	120	32	0	32	0	0
Apple slices	1 svg	100	26	5	21	1	0
Applesauce	1 svg	110	27	1	26	0	0
Bacon	2 pc	70	0	0	0	6	6

	SERVING SIZE	CALORIES	TOTAL CARBS (g)	FIBER (g)	NET CARBS (g)	PROTEIN (g)	FAT (g)
Friendly's (cont.)	...	...	.	.	.	.	.
Bacon	3 pc	110	0	0	0	8	8
Bacon	4 pc	140	0	0	0	11	11
Bacon cheese supermelt, w/o potatoes	1	680	52	3	49	33	39
Bacon cheeseburger	1	940	55	3	52	43	61
Bagel	1	350	55	5	50	10	11
Bagel w/ cream cheese	1	440	57	5	52	11	19
Balsamic vinaigrette dressing	1 svg	180	9	0	9	0	15
Balsamic vinaigrette dressing, side salad	1 svg	90	5	0	5	0	8
Banana	1	40	9	0	9	0	0
Banana smoothie	1	520	104	1	103	17	4
Barq's float	1	580	98	0	98	6	19
BBQ chicken platter	1	1010	75	2	73	79	42
BBQ chicken, 2+2	1	590	46	2	44	41	26
BBQ sauce	1 svg	90	20	0	20	0	0
Birthday cake Friend-z	1	690	100	0	100	9	29
Black raspberry ice cream	1 scoop	120	15	0	15	2	5
Bleu cheese dressing, side salad	1 svg	240	2	0	2	3	24
Blue cheese dressing	1 svg	470	3	0	3	6	48
Blueberry muffin	1	610	64	1	63	7	36

	SERVING SIZE	CALORIES	TOTAL CARBS (g)	FIBER (g)	NET CARBS (g)	PROTEIN (g)	FAT (g)
Friendly's (cont.)	...	...	.	.	.	.	.
Broccoli	1 svg	90	6	4	2	3	6
Broccoli cheddar soup	1 cup	170	10	1	9	6	12
Broccoli cheddar soup	1 bowl	340	20	2	18	12	24
Buffalo chicken	1	1200	45	5	40	41	95
Buffalo chicken sandwich	1	940	69	6	63	30	61
Buffalo chicken wrap	1	1180	75	5	70	38	80
Butter crunch ice cream	1 scoop	130	16	0	16	2	6
Butter pecan ice cream	1 scoop	130	13	0	13	2	8
Butterfinger pieces topping	1 svg	120	18	1	17	1	5
Butterfinger sundae	1	830	117	2	115	9	36
Cake cone	1	30	7	0	7	1	0
Caramel fudge brownie sundae	1	1410	186	2	184	19	66
Caramel topping	1 svg	130	27	0	27	1	2
Cereal, *Froot Loops*	1 svg	250	46	1	45	8	3
Cereal, *Raisin Bran Crunch*	1 svg	370	77	6	71	11	3
Cheddar jack chicken	1	640	5	1	4	78	34
Cheddar jack chicken, 2+2	1	320	3	1	2	39	17
Cherry	1	10	2	0	2	0	0
Chicken Caesar salad, w/dressing	1	1030	32	3	29	47	84

	SERVING SIZE	CALORIES	TOTAL CARBS (g)	FIBER (g)	NET CARBS (g)	PROTEIN (g)	FAT (g)
Friendly's (cont.)	. . .	. . .	.	.	.	.	.
Chicken deluxe sandwich, side bacon	1	70	0	0	0	6	6
Chicken deluxe sandwich, side cheese	1	90	1	0	1	4	7
Chicken fajita quesadilla	1	1220	65	7	58	67	77
Chicken parm supermelt	1	830	73	4	69	43	43
Chicken quesadilla	1	570	29	3	26	33	35
Chicken quesadilla	1	1020	56	4	52	29	67
Chicken strips basket	6 pc	650	39	3	36	39	38
Chicken strips basket	5 pc	540	32	3	29	32	32
Chocolate almond chip ice cream	1 scoop	120	11	0	11	2	7
Chocolate chip cookie dough ice cream	1 scoop	130	17	0	17	2	7
Chocolate chip ice cream	1 scoop	130	15	0	15	2	7
Chocolate ice cream	1 scoop	110	10	0	10	2	6
Chocolate soft serve	4 oz	170	24	0	24	4	6
Chocolate soft serve	8 oz	340	49	0	49	9	12
Chocolate sprinkles	1 svg	120	19	0	19	0	5
Chocolate syrup topping	1 svg	100	23	1	22	1	0

	SERVING SIZE	CALORIES	TOTAL CARBS (g)	FIBER (g)	NET CARBS (g)	PROTEIN (g)	FAT (g)
Friendly's (cont.)	...	...	.	.	.	.	.
Chunky chicken noodle soup	1 cup	260	27	2	25	19	9
Chunky chicken noodle soup	1 bowl	510	54	3	51	38	17
Clamboat basket	1	990	104	6	98	24	54
Cocktail sauce	1 svg	30	8	0	8	1	0
Coffee ice cream	1 scoop	110	13	0	13	2	6
Cole slaw	1 svg	160	13	2	11	1	12
Colossal burger	1	1490	56	4	52	82	104
Cookies 'n cream ice cream	1 scoop	130	16	0	16	2	6
Corn	1 svg	160	20	4	16	4	7
Country club chicken sandwich	1	940	71	6	65	40	57
Cranberry juice, large	1	250	62	0	62	0	0
Cranberry juice, small	1	150	37	0	37	0	0
Cranberry muffin	1	630	59	2	57	8	40
Crispy chicken Caesar wrap	1	1180	75	5	70	40	80
Crispy chicken salad	1	710	45	6	39	37	42
Crispy chicken tender deluxe sandwich	1	800	72	6	66	28	46
Crispy chicken wrap	1	800	84	6	78	27	40
Crushed *Heath* topping	1 svg	170	19	0	19	1	10
Crushed *Oreo* topping	1 svg	60	9	0	9	1	2

	SERVING SIZE	CALORIES	TOTAL CARBS (g)	FIBER (g)	NET CARBS (g)	PROTEIN (g)	FAT (g)
Friendly's (cont.)	...	...	.	.	.	.	.
Deluxe cheeseburger "set-up"	1	850	35	3	32	40	61
Double thick milkshake, chocolate	1	700	85	1	84	21	32
Double thick milkshake, coffee	1	770	107	0	107	15	32
Double thick milkshake, strawberry	1	740	110	0	110	16	27
Double thick milkshake, vanilla	1	770	106	0	106	15	32
Eggbeaters, scrambled	1	50	1	0	1	8	3
Eggbeaters, scrambled	2	100	1	0	1	16	5
Eggbeaters, scrambled	3	160	2	0	2	24	8
Eggs, poached	1	70	0	0	0	6	5
Eggs, poached	2	140	1	0	1	13	10
Eggs, poached	3	210	1	0	1	19	15
Eggs, scrambled	1	110	1	0	1	7	8
Eggs, scrambled	2	220	3	0	3	14	16
Eggs, scrambled	3	320	4	0	4	21	25
Eggs, sunny-side up	1	90	0	0	0	6	7
Eggs, sunny-side up	2	180	1	0	1	13	14
Eggs, sunny-side up	3	270	1	0	1	19	21
English muffin	1	310	45	2	43	8	11
Fat-free Italian dressing, side salad	1 svg	30	8	0	8	0	0
Fishamajig	1	640	51	3	48	26	37

	SERVING SIZE	CALORIES	TOTAL CARBS (g)	FIBER (g)	NET CARBS (g)	PROTEIN (g)	FAT (g)
Friendly's (cont.)	...	...	.	.	.	.	.
Forbidden chocolate ice cream	1 scoop	130	14	0	14	3	7
Forbidden fudge brownie	1	940	131	4	127	13	41
Four cheese & bacon omelette, w/o potatoes or toast	1	670	8	0	8	46	50
French toast	3 pc	760	128	3	125	16	20
Fribble shake, *Butterfinger*	1	990	155	2	153	19	33
Fribble shake, chocolate	1	590	94	1	93	19	17
Fribble shake, coffee	1	630	102	0	102	16	19
Fribble shake, strawberry	1	610	93	0	93	16	19
Fribble shake, vanilla	1	620	100	0	100	16	19
Fried shrimp, 2+2	1	330	32	2	30	12	17
Friendly frank	1	410	25	1	24	11	30
Friendly's BLT	1	680	51	3	48	20	45
Friend-z *Butterfinger*	1	820	122	3	119	11	32
Friend-z *Heath*	1	680	88	0	88	9	34
Friend-z *Kit Kat*	1	690	93	1	92	11	31
Friend-z *M&M*	1	560	80	2	78	10	23
Friend-z *Oreo*	1	580	84	2	82	9	23
Friend-z *Reese's* Peanut Butter Cup	1	860	96	4	92	20	45
Friend-z *Strawberry* shortcake	1	470	72	1	71	8	17

	SERVING SIZE	CALORIES	TOTAL CARBS (g)	FIBER (g)	NET CARBS (g)	PROTEIN (g)	FAT (g)
Friendly's (cont.)	...	...	.	.	.	.	.
Friend-z strawberry/ banana	1	430	69	1	68	8	14
Fruit & sherbet happy ending sundae	1	240	47	0	47	2	5
Fudge topping, no sugar added	1 svg	90	25	2	23	1	0
Garden omelette, w/o potatoes or toast	1	860	52	5	47	40	55
Garden vegetables	1 svg	110	13	4	9	3	6
Garlic bread	1 svg	130	18	0	18	3	6
Giant crowd pleaser	1	2480	317	4	313	41	118
Golden fries	1 svg	300	44	4	40	3	13
Grape jelly	1 svg	60	14	0	14	0	0
Grapefruit juice, large	1	190	45	0	45	4	0
Grapefruit juice, small	1	120	27	0	27	2	0
Grilled cheese	1	460	48	2	46	16	23
Grilled chicken deluxe sandwich	1	640	54	5	49	38	32
Grilled flounder	1	520	28	2	26	29	32
Grilled flounder, 2+2	1	260	15	2	13	15	16
Grilled ham & cheese	1	510	49	2	47	28	23
Gummy bear topping	1 svg	90	21	0	21	1	0
Ham & cheese omelette, w/o potatoes or toast	1	580	9	0	9	50	43

	SERVING SIZE	CALORIES	TOTAL CARBS (g)	FIBER (g)	NET CARBS (g)	PROTEIN (g)	FAT (g)
Friendly's (cont.)	...	...	.	.	.	.	.
Ham & cheese supermelt, w/o potatoes	1	660	53	3	50	34	35
Hickory smoked ham	1 pc	100	2	0	2	14	4
Homefries	1 svg	290	41	4	37	5	12
Homestyle clam chowder	1 cup	240	13	1	12	10	17
Homestyle clam chowder	1 bowl	490	26	1	25	20	35
Homestyle mashed potatoes	1 svg	240	29	2	27	4	12
Homestyle meatloaf	1	850	45	1	44	54	49
Honey BBQ chicken strips	6 pc	1020	133	3	130	39	38
Honey BBQ chicken strips	5 pc	910	126	3	123	32	32
Honey BBQ chicken supermelt	1	1080	86	4	82	47	62
Honey BBQ sauce	1 svg	180	12	0	12	0	15
Honey mustard chicken sandwich	1	850	74	6	68	33	49
Honey mustard dressing	1 svg	360	24	0	24	0	30
Honey mustard dressing, side salad	1 svg	180	12	0	12	0	15
Hot fudge topping	1 svg	120	19	0	19	2	4
Hunka chunka fudge ice cream	1 scoop	180	17	1	16	3	11
Italian dressing	1 svg	410	6	0	6	0	42
Italian dressing, side salad	1 svg	210	3	0	3	0	21

	SERVING SIZE	CALORIES	TOTAL CARBS (g)	FIBER (g)	NET CARBS (g)	PROTEIN (g)	FAT (g)
Friendly's (cont.)	...	...	.	.	.	.	.
Jim dandy	1	1090	156	2	154	14	47
Jumbo fronions & waffle fries	1	1270	134	8	126	12	76
Kickin' buffalo chicken salad	1	770	48	6	42	31	50
Kickin' buffalo chicken strips	6 pc	910	42	3	39	39	65
Kickin' buffalo chicken strips	5 pc	810	35	3	32	32	59
Kit Kat bar topping	1 svg	80	11	0	11	1	4
Kit Kat sundae	1	740	91	1	90	10	37
Loaded waffle fries	1	1660	123	9	114	32	112
Loaded jumbo fronions & waffle fries	1	1600	129	8	121	23	110
M&M's topping	1 svg	100	15	1	14	1	5
Malt powder, add on	1 svg	90	15	0	15	2	2
Mandarin oranges	1 svg	80	20	0	20	0	0
Maple walnut ice cream	1 scoop	130	13	0	13	2	8
Marshmallow topping	1 svg	100	24	0	24	0	0
Minestrone soup	1 cup	60	11	2	9	3	1
Minestrone soup	1 bowl	120	23	5	18	6	2
Mini mozzarella cheese sticks	1	680	55	4	51	24	40
Mint chocolate ice cream	1 scoop	130	15	0	15	2	7
Mocha mud crunch ice cream	1 scoop	160	18	1	17	2	9
Munchie Mania	1	1670	123	8	115	52	108
Mushroom swiss bacon burger	1	1240	61	3	58	59	87

	SERVING SIZE	CALORIES	TOTAL CARBS (g)	FIBER (g)	NET CARBS (g)	PROTEIN (g)	FAT (g)
Friendly's (cont.)	...	...	.	.	.	.	.
New England fish 'n chips	1	660	45	3	42	21	44
Non-fat red raspberry swirl yogurt	1 scoop	90	19	0	19	3	0
Non-fat vanilla yogurt	1 scoop	80	17	0	17	3	0
Nuts over caramel ice cream	1 scoop	150	18	0	18	2	8
Orange juice, large	1	210	49	0	49	4	0
Orange juice, small	1	130	29	0	29	2	0
Orange marmalade	1 svg	40	10	0	10	0	0
Orange sherbet ice cream	1 scoop	80	17	0	17	1	1
Orange slammer	1	600	138	0	138	3	4
Oreo freeze	1	770	120	2	118	18	25
Oriental chicken salad	1	500	41	5	36	37	21
Pancake syrup	1 svg	240	58	0	58	0	0
Pancakes	3	930	175	5	170	14	17
Pancakes	2	500	77	3	74	9	17
Peanut butter cup ice cream	1 scoop	150	16	1	15	3	9
Peanut butter cup topping	1 svg	90	10	1	9	2	5
Peanut butter topping	1 svg	210	7	3	4	7	17
Pineapple smoothie	1	590	122	1	121	16	4
Pistachio ice cream	1 scoop	130	14	0	14	3	7
Popcorn chicken	1	610	46	3	43	38	30
Rainbow sprinkles	1 svg	120	18	0	18	0	5
Ranch dressing	1 svg	330	3	0	3	3	33

	SERVING SIZE	CALORIES	TOTAL CARBS (g)	FIBER (g)	NET CARBS (g)	PROTEIN (g)	FAT (g)
Friendly's (cont.)	...	...	.	.	.	.	.
Ranch dressing, side salad	1 svg	160	2	0	2	2	17
Reese's Peanut Butter Cup sundae	1	890	90	7	83	17	52
Reese's Pieces sundae	1	640	152	4	148	23	71
Reese's pieces topping	1 svg	130	15	1	14	3	6
Reuben supermelt	1	800	57	2	55	50	42
Rice	1 svg	210	41	0	41	3	3
Roasted sliced almond topping	1 svg	110	3	2	1	4	10
Royal banana split	1	880	132	2	130	10	35
Saltine crackers	1 pkt	30	4	0	4	1	1
Sausage	2	200	0	0	0	6	19
Sausage	3	300	1	0	1	9	29
Sausage	4	390	1	0	1	12	38
Sausage mushroom swiss supermelt, w/o potatoes	1	910	56	4	52	42	58
Sesame oriental dressing	1 svg	270	36	0	36	0	14
Sesame oriental dressing, side salad	1 svg	130	18	0	18	0	7
Shrimp basket	1	570	42	4	38	21	35
Side Caesar salad, w/ dressing	1	410	15	1	14	9	36
Side salad	1	60	10	2	8	2	1
Sirloin steak	1	510	19	1	18	46	28
Sirloin steak tips	1	490	31	5	26	46	20

	SERVING SIZE	CALORIES	TOTAL CARBS (g)	FIBER (g)	NET CARBS (g)	PROTEIN (g)	FAT (g)
Friendly's (cont.)	...	...	.	.	.	.	.
Sirloin steak tips, 2+2	1	490	31	5	26	46	20
Sirloin steak, 2+2	1	510	19	1	18	46	28
Slider munchie mania, chicken	1	1990	161	14	147	52	127
Slider munchie mania, mini cheeseburger	1	1740	141	12	129	49	109
Southwest BBQ steak	1	760	37	2	35	57	42
Southwest BBQ steak, 2+2	1	750	37	1	36	57	42
Spanish rice	1 svg	330	41	0	41	7	15
Strawberry banana smoothie	1	520	105	2	103	17	4
Strawberry ice cream	1 scoop	110	14	0	14	2	5
Strawberry shortcake sundae	1	580	79	2	77	8	27
Strawberry topping	1 svg	190	48	4	44	1	0
Sugar cone	1	50	11	0	11	1	0
Super sizzlin bacon, w/o eggs & toast	1	440	42	4	38	16	23
Super sizzlin ham, w/o eggs & toast	1	450	45	4	41	26	18
Super sizzlin sausage, w/o eggs & toast	1	690	43	4	39	17	50
Super sizzlin/ combo, w/o eggs & toast	1	570	43	4	39	16	37
Swiss chocolate topping	1 svg	100	25	0	25	0	0

	SERVING SIZE	CALORIES	TOTAL CARBS (g)	FIBER (g)	NET CARBS (g)	PROTEIN (g)	FAT (g)
Friendly's (cont.)	...	...	.	.	.	.	.
Swiss patty melt	1	1030	62	4	58	52	64
Tartar sauce	1 svg	230	6	0	6	0	23
Thousand island dressing	1 svg	390	15	0	15	0	36
Thousand island dressing, side salad	1 svg	190	8	0	8	0	18
Toast, rye	1	340	48	2	46	10	12
Toast, wheat	1	200	22	2	20	5	10
Toast, white	1	200	23	2	21	4	10
Tomato juice, large	1	90	19	4	15	4	0
Tomato juice, small	1	60	11	2	9	2	0
Towering fronions	1	1430	140	7	133	14	90
Tri-tip steak	1 pc	350	0	0	0	44	19
Tuna roll	1	580	25	2	23	24	43
Tuna supermelt	1	810	50	3	47	35	52
Turkey burger	1	1140	61	3	58	50	78
Turkey club supermelt	1	670	54	3	51	42	33
Twist soft serve	4 oz	170	25	0	25	4	7
Twist soft serve	8 oz	350	50	0	50	8	13
Ultimate bacon cheeseburger	1	1050	55	3	52	52	69
Ultimate cookies & cream	1	690	86	1	85	11	33
Vanilla ice cream	1 scoop	120	14	0	14	2	6
Vanilla ice cream, no sugar added	1 scoop	100	11	3	8	2	7
Vanilla soft serve	4 oz	180	25	0	25	3	7
Vanilla soft serve	8 oz	360	51	0	51	7	14
Vegetable fajita quesadilla	1	1210	77	12	65	43	82

	SERVING SIZE	CALORIES	TOTAL CARBS (g)	FIBER (g)	NET CARBS (g)	PROTEIN (g)	FAT (g)
Friendly's (cont.)	...	...	.	.	.	.	.
Vienna mocha chunk ice cream	1 scoop	140	16	0	16	2	8
Waffle cone	1	90	20	1	19	2	1
Waffle fries	1 svg	590	67	5	62	7	33
Walnut topping	1 svg	100	2	0	2	0	10
Watermelon sherbet	1 scoop	80	17	0	17	1	1
Watermelon slammer	1	450	100	0	100	3	4
Western BBQ burger	1	1230	86	4	82	51	77
Western omelette, w/o potatoes or toast	1	640	12	1	11	45	45
Whipped topping	1 svg	80	5	0	5	1	6
Jason's Deli	...	...	.	.	.	.	.
American potato salad	8 oz	420	32	4	28	6	29
Amy's turkey-o sandwich	1	650	71	7	64	33	27
Baklava	1	380	50	2	48	6	16
Beefeater po'boy	1	790	41	1	40	64	38
Big chef salad	1	550	25	7	18	53	28
Bird to the wise w/ mayo	1	1490	49	0	49	71	113
Bird to the wise, no dressing	1	1390	49	0	49	71	102
BLT	1	800	68	10	58	30	49
Broccoli cheese soup	12 oz	450	27	2	25	19	30
Bronx baker potato	1	860	132	14	118	28	26
Caesar salad w/ bread	1	1220	68	6	62	30	93

	SERVING SIZE	CALORIES	TOTAL CARBS (g)	FIBER (g)	NET CARBS (g)	PROTEIN (g)	FAT (g)
Jason's Deli (cont.)	...	...	.	.	.	.	.
Caesar salad, side	1	660	53	6	47	16	43
Café wrap	1	780	38	4	34	49	50
California club sandwich	1	830	42	2	40	39	57
Cantina wrapini	1	690	57	17	40	55	35
Carrot cake	1	510	63	4	59	6	28
Chicken pasta primo, w/ bread	1	990	68	5	63	50	61
Cheese cake, fruit topped	1	570	61	1	60	8	34
Cheese cake, plain	1	520	54	1	53	9	31
Cheese cake, strawberry	1	530	56	1	55	5	31
Cheese cake, triple chocolate	1	550	58	2	56	8	32
Cheese cake, turtle	1	500	50	2	48	8	30
Chicago club sandwich	1	780	46	7	39	46	50
Chicken Caesar salad w/ bread	1	1400	72	6	66	61	99
Chicken club wrapini	1	780	42	4	38	56	46
Chicken noodle soup	12 oz	210	24	2	22	12	8
Chicken panini	1	840	49	2	47	53	48
Chicken pasta alfredo, w/bread	1	1200	68	3	65	58	80
Chicken pot pie, w/ pastry	12 oz	450	45	3	42	17	23
Chocolate chip cookie	1	330	40	Tr	40	4	18
Chocolate soft serve dessert	1	170	25	0	25	5	5

	SERVING SIZE	CALORIES	TOTAL CARBS (g)	FIBER (g)	NET CARBS (g)	PROTEIN (g)	FAT (g)
Jason's Deli (cont.)	...	...	.	.	.	.	.
Chocolate topping, for ice cream	1 oz	100	22	1	21	1	1
Ciabatta bing sandwich	1	520	60	11	49	30	19
Ciabatta garden sandwich	1	420	50	7	43	16	19
Clam chowder	12 oz	300	21	1	20	10	20
Club lite	1	510	50	6	44	43	16
Club royale sandwich	1	850	44	2	42	53	51
Cranberry walnut cookie	1	310	39	3	36	5	16
Creamy fruit dip	1	60	8	0	8	1	3
Creamy Irish potato soup	12 oz	460	33	2	31	8	33
Deli club sandwich	1	880	70	9	61	58	44
Deli cowboy po'boy	1	830	66	2	64	70	47
Dill pickle spear	1 oz	5	1	1	0	0	0
Fire roasted tortilla soup	12 oz	320	35	5	30	9	16
Fresh fruit cup	1	230	41	3	38	3	8
Fresh fruit cup, no dip	1	90	23	3	20	1	0
Fresh fruit plate	1	390	78	8	70	7	9
Fresh fruit plate, no dip	1	240	61	8	53	5	1
Fudge nut brownie	1	420	51	3	48	6	24
Garlic olive oil foccacia bread, for caesar salad	1	400	37	2	35	7	27
Garlic olive oil foccacia bread, side	2 pc	400	37	2	35	7	27

	SERVING SIZE	CALORIES	TOTAL CARBS (g)	FIBER (g)	NET CARBS (g)	PROTEIN (g)	FAT (g)
Jason's Deli (cont.)	. . .	. . .	.	.	.	.	.
Grilled portobello wrapini	1	670	45	7	38	24	47
Guacamole	4 oz	170	10	7	3	2	15
Ham muffaletta, ½	1	870	71	7	64	52	41
Ham muffaletta, ¼	1	440	36	3	33	26	21
Ham muffaletta, whole	1	1750	142	13	129	105	83
Ham panini	1	470	46	2	44	24	20
Hamit down sandwich	1	460	49	2	47	40	11
Homemade salsa	4 oz	30	7	2	5	1	0
Honeymustard coleslaw	8 oz	190	25	4	21	4	9
House chips	1 oz	230	22	1	21	3	15
Ice cream cone	1	20	4	0	4	0	0
Italian pasta salad	8 oz	720	106	6	100	20	25
JB's bagelini	1	620	50	5	45	28	35
Low fat fruit & yogurt parfait cup	1	230	43	2	41	9	3
Macadamia white chip cookie	1	340	39	Tr	39	4	18
Marinated chicken breast salad	1	580	32	10	22	52	30
Mario's big cheesy sandwich	1	700	58	15	43	33	42
Meatabella po'boy	1	1070	62	3	59	52	65
Mediterranean wrap	1	310	43	6	37	14	10
Miami panini	1	570	44	2	42	49	21
Nutty mixed up salad	1	920	93	9	84	36	45
Nutty mixed up salad w/o chicken	1	740	87	9	78	10	40

	SERVING SIZE	CALORIES	TOTAL CARBS (g)	FIBER (g)	NET CARBS (g)	PROTEIN (g)	FAT (g)
Jason's Deli (cont.)	...	...	.	.	.	.	.
Nutty mixed up salad w/o chicken & dressing	1	460	77	8	69	10	12
Nutty mixed up salad w/o dressing	1	640	80	8	72	41	18
Oatmeal cookie	1	270	48	2	46	4	7
Organic blue corn tortilla chips	1 oz	210	26	3	23	3	11
Pasta alfredo, w/bread	1	1020	65	3	62	28	74
Pasta primo, w/bread	1	800	64	5	59	18	54
Pastrami melt po'boy	1	1230	44	1	43	50	94
Peanut butter cookie	1	340	34	2	32	7	20
Penne pasta w/ meatballs, w/ bread	1	1110	74	5	69	40	74
Philly chic sandwich	1	610	52	5	47	47	25
Pizza adobe	1	740	49	3	46	48	41
Pizza blue	1	850	35	10	25	37	65
Plain Jane potato	1	2300	190	13	177	60	147
Poblano corn chowder	12 oz	340	38	4	34	8	19
Pollo Mexicano potato	1	1760	200	16	184	65	81
Portobello garden pasta w/ chicken, w/ bread	1	1120	76	12	64	57	69

	SERVING SIZE	CALORIES	TOTAL CARBS (g)	FIBER (g)	NET CARBS (g)	PROTEIN (g)	FAT (g)
Jason's Deli (cont.)	. . .	. . .	.	.	.	.	.
Portobello garden pasta w/ mushrooms, w/ bread	1	950	74	12	62	26	63
Pot roast melt po'boy	1	770	47	4	43	67	32
Pulled pork sandwich, onion bun	1	660	74	2	72	43	22
Pulled pork sandwich, wheat bun	1	710	83	2	81	44	23
Ranchero wrap	1	890	62	13	49	61	49
Red beans & rice w/ sausage	12 oz	280	56	23	33	19	6
Reuben the great sandwich	1	860	56	9	47	75	35
Roasted red pepper hummus	4 oz	240	28	8	20	8	14
Santa Fe chicken sandwich	1	760	52	7	45	57	38
Seafood gumbo	12 oz	300	37	3	34	16	10
Sergeant pepper po'boy	1	900	52	4	48	66	43
Smokey Jack melt	1	590	53	5	48	42	25
Smokey Jack panini	1	790	52	3	49	50	42
Spinach veggie wrap	1	360	40	6	34	16	17
Spud au broc	1	1540	203	17	186	68	56
Steamed veggies	1	60	13	5	8	4	0
Strawberry short cake	1	410	63	1	62	6	15

	SERVING SIZE	CALORIES	TOTAL CARBS (g)	FIBER (g)	NET CARBS (g)	PROTEIN (g)	FAT (g)
Jason's Deli (cont.)	...	...	.	.	.	.	.
SW chicken chili, plain	12 oz	270	27	7	20	25	9
Taco salad w/ chili	1	1970	189	27	162	55	111
Taco salad w/ SW chicken chili	1	1910	193	28	165	49	105
Texas chili	12 oz	400	20	6	14	35	20
Texas style spud w/ beef	1	1640	189	13	176	46	75
Texas style spud w/ pork	1	1550	191	13	178	48	68
The italian Cruz po'boy	1	650	50	4	46	32	35
The New York Yankee sandwich, no dressing	1	1190	47	2	45	92	69
The VJ sandwich, no dressing	1	890	37	2	35	58	57
The VJ sandwich, w/ mayo	1	990	37	2	35	58	68
The VJ sandwich, w/ mustard	1	910	37	2	35	58	57
Three bean salad	8 oz	400	41	12	29	22	14
Tomato basil soup	12 oz	320	22	4	18	3	25
Tuna & roasted tomato wrap	1	560	59	11	48	22	27
Tuna melt	1	960	47	6	41	54	62
Tuna pasta salad	8 oz	590	67	4	63	23	27
Turkey muffaletta, 1/2	1	780	73	7	66	52	32
Turkey muffaletta, 1/4	1	390	37	3	34	26	16
Turkey muffaletta, whole	1	1560	146	13	133	103	64

	SERVING SIZE	CALORIES	TOTAL CARBS (g)	FIBER (g)	NET CARBS (g)	PROTEIN (g)	FAT (g)
Jason's Deli (cont.)	. . .	. . .	.	.	.	.	.
Turkey reuben sandwich	1	510	53	6	47	44	13
Turkey wrap	1	360	40	5	35	22	14
Twisted turkey salad w/ dressing	1	1020	48	13	35	52	68
Twisted turkey salad w/o dressing	1	860	28	13	15	52	60
Uptown turkey melt	1	400	28	3	25	38	16
Vanilla soft serve dessert	1	160	24	0	24	3	5
Vegetarian French onion soup, w/ bread & cheese	12 oz	270	17	1	16	9	19
Vegetarian vegetable pasta soup	12 oz	130	23	4	19	3	3
Hardees	. . .	. . .	.	.	.	.	.
Apple turnover	1	290	36	1	35	2	15
Bacon cheese Thickburger	1	850	49	3	46	38	57
Bacon, egg & cheese biscuit	1	530	36	0	36	15	36
BBQ chicken sandwich	1	400	62	5	57	27	6
Big chicken fillet sandwich	1	710	62	5	57	33	38
Big country breakfast platter w/ bacon	1	910	91	4	87	27	48
Big roast beef sandwich	1	400	28	1	27	25	21
Biscuit "n" gravy	1	530	48	1	47	9	33

	SERVING SIZE	CALORIES	TOTAL CARBS (g)	FIBER (g)	NET CARBS (g)	PROTEIN (g)	FAT (g)
Hardees (cont.)	...	...	.	.	.	.	.
Breaded pork chop biscuit	1	640	46	1	45	25	39
Charbroiled chicken club sandwich	1	630	54	4	50	32	32
Cheeseburger	1	620	51	3	48	35	33
Chicken fillet biscuit	1	600	50	1	49	24	34
Chicken strips	3 pc	370	19	2	17	14	26
Chicken strips	5 pc	610	32	3	29	23	43
Chocolate cake	1 svg	300	56	2	54	4	12
Chocolate chip cookie	1	290	44	0	44	4	11
Chocolate chip cookie, fresh baked	1	250	30	1	29	2	14
Cinnamon "n" raisin biscuit	1	300	40	1	39	3	15
Cole slaw, small	1 svg	170	20	2	18	1	10
Country ham biscuit	1	440	36	0	36	14	26
Country potatoes, medium	1	290	39	4	35	6	12
Country steak biscuit	1	630	45	0	45	16	43
Crispy curls, medium	1	410	52	4	48	5	20
Double bacon cheese Thickburger	1	1200	50	3	47	65	84
Double cheeseburger	1	530	34	1	33	27	32
Double Thickburger	1	1150	53	2	51	62	78

	SERVING SIZE	CALORIES	TOTAL CARBS (g)	FIBER (g)	NET CARBS (g)	PROTEIN (g)	FAT (g)
Hardees (cont.)	...	...	.	.	.	.	.
Fish supreme sandwich	1	630	51	3	48	22	38
French fries, large	1	470	65	5	61	5	21
French fries, medium	1	430	60	4	56	5	19
French fries, small	1	320	45	3	42	4	14
Fried chicken breast	1	370	29	0	29	29	15
Fried chicken leg	1	170	15	0	15	13	7
Fried chicken thigh	1	330	30	0	30	19	15
Fried chicken wing	1	200	23	0	23	10	8
Frisco breakfast sandwich	1	400	27	2	25	23	18
Grits	1 svg	110	16	1	15	2	5
Ham, egg, & cheese biscuit	1	540	36	0	36	23	33
Hand-scooped malt	1	780	98	0	98	17	35
Hand-scooped shake	1	705	86	0	86	14	33
Hot ham "n" cheese sandwich	1	460	40	2	38	36	20
Jelly biscuit	1	520	44	0	44	5	34
Jumbo chili dog	1	400	25	1	24	16	26
Little Thick cheeseburger	1	450	38	3	35	24	23
Little Thickburger	1	570	35	3	32	24	39
Loaded biscuit "n" gravy breakfast bowl	1	740	49	1	48	20	52
Loaded breakfast burrito	1	760	39	1	38	39	49
Loaded omelet biscuit	1	610	36	0	36	20	42

	SERVING SIZE	CALORIES	TOTAL CARBS (g)	FIBER (g)	NET CARBS (g)	PROTEIN (g)	FAT (g)
Hardees (cont.)	. . .	. . .	.	.	.	.	.
Low-carb breakfast bowl	1	620	6	2	4	36	50
Low-carb charbroiled chicken club sandwich	1	360	14	1	13	24	23
Low-carb Thickburger	1	420	5	2	3	30	32
Made from scratch biscuit	1	370	35	0	35	5	23
Mashed potatoes, small	1 svg	90	17	0	17	1	2
Monster biscuit	1	770	37	0	37	29	55
Monster Thickburger	1	1320	46	2	44	70	95
Mushroom & swiss Thickburger	1	650	47	3	44	39	36
Original Thickburger	1	770	53	4	49	35	48
Pancakes, 3 per svg	1 svg	300	55	2	53	8	5
Peach cobbler, sm	1 svg	290	56	1	55	1	7
Pork chop "n" gravy biscuit	1	680	48	1	47	26	42
Regular roast beef sandwich	1	310	28	1	27	17	15
Sausage & egg biscuit	1	590	36	0	36	16	42
Sausage biscuit	1	530	36	0	36	11	38
Side salad, w/o dressing	1	120	7	2	5	7	7
Single scoop ice cream bowl	1	235	27	0	27	5	13

	SERVING SIZE	CALORIES	TOTAL CARBS (g)	FIBER (g)	NET CARBS (g)	PROTEIN (g)	FAT (g)
Hardees (cont.)	...	...	.	.	.	.	.
Single scoop ice cream cone	1	285	37	0	37	6	13
Six Dollar Thickburger	1	930	57	4	53	46	59
Small cheeseburger	1	350	32	1	31	16	19
Small hamburger	1	310	32	1	31	14	15
Smoked sausage biscuit	1	620	37	0	37	14	46
Spicy chicken sandwich	1	440	41	3	38	11	21
Sunrise croissant w/ ham	1	400	27	1	26	21	23
In-N-Out Burger	...	...	.	.	.	.	.
Cheeseburger w/ onion, ketchup & mustard	1	400	41	3	38	22	18
Cheeseburger w/ onion, spread	1	480	39	3	36	22	27
Cheeseburger w/ onion, Protein style (lettuce, no bun)	1	330	11	3	8	18	25
Chocolate shake	15 oz	690	83	0	83	9	36
Double-Double w/ onion, ketchup & mustard	1	590	41	3	38	37	32
Double-Double w/ onion, spread	1	670	39	3	36	37	41
Double-Double w/ onion, Protein style (lettuce, no bun)	1	520	11	3	8	33	39
French fries	1 svg	400	54	2	52	7	18

	SERVING SIZE	CALORIES	TOTAL CARBS (g)	FIBER (g)	NET CARBS (g)	PROTEIN (g)	FAT (g)
In–N–Out Burger	...	...	.	.	.	.	.
(cont.)							
Hamburger w/ onion, ketchup & mustard	1	310	41	3	38	16	10
Hamburger w/ onion, spread	1	390	39	3	36	16	19
Hamburger w/ onion, Protein style (lettuce, no bun)	1	240	11	3	8	13	17
Lemonade	16 oz	180	40	0	40	0	0
Minute Maid Light Lemonade	16 oz	10	1	0	1	0	0
Strawberry shake	15 oz	690	91	0	91	9	33
Vanilla shake	15 oz	680	78	0	78	9	37
Jack-In-The-Box	...	...	.	.	.	.	.
Asian Chicken Salad w/ Crispy Chicken	1	340	38	8	30	21	13
Asian Chicken Salad w/ Grilled Chicken	1	180	22	6	16	22	2
Asian Sesame Dressing	1 svg	190	16	0	16	1	14
Bacon, Egg & Cheese Biscuit	1	440	37	2	35	15	25
Bacon Ranch Dressing	1 svg	260	3	0	3	2	26
Beef Taco	1	160	190	15	175	5	70
Breakfast Jack	1	290	29	1	28	16	12
Breakfast sandwich, sourdough	1	440	37	2	35	19	24
Burger, Sirloin – Mini	1	750	77	3	74	42	29

	SERVING SIZE	CALORIES	TOTAL CARBS (g)	FIBER (g)	NET CARBS (g)	PROTEIN (g)	FAT (g)
Jack-In-The-Box	...	...	.	.	.	.	.
(cont.)							
Burger, Sirloin, Swiss & Grilled Onions	1	930	60	4	56	42	59
Burger, Sirloin, Swiss & Grilled onions w/ bacon	1	990	61	4	57	47	64
Cheeseburger, Big	1	650	50	2	48	24	40
Cheeseburger, Junior Bacon	1	400	30	1	29	18	23
Cheeseburger, Sirloin	1	950	61	4	57	41	60
Cheeseburger, Sirloin, w/ Bacon	1	1010	62	4	58	46	65
Cheeseburger, Ultimate	1	920	52	2	50	38	63
Cheeseburger, Ultimate w/ bacon	1	980	52	2	50	43	67
Cheesecake	1 pc	310	34	0	34	7	16
Chicken Breast Strips (4), crispy	1 svg	500	36	3	33	35	25
Chicken Breast Strips (4), grilled	1 svg	180	3	0	3	37	19
Chicken Club Salad w/ Crispy Chicken	1	480	28	6	22	33	27
Chicken Club Salad w/ Grilled Chicken	1	320	12	4	8	34	16
Chicken Fajita Pita, whole grain, no sauce	1	320	33	4	29	24	11
Chicken Sandwich	1	400	38	2	36	15	21
Chicken Sandwich w/ bacon	1	440	38	2	36	19	24

	SERVING SIZE	CALORIES	TOTAL CARBS (g)	FIBER (g)	NET CARBS (g)	PROTEIN (g)	FAT (g)
Jack-In-The-Box	...	...	.	.	.	.	.
(cont.)							
Chocolate Overload Cake	1 svg	300	57	2	55	4	60
Chorizo Sausage Burrito	1	700	59	6	53	28	38
Creamy Southwest Dressing	1 svg	470	44	9	35	30	23
Denver Breakfast Burrito	1	720	36	5	31	26	53
Egg roll	1	130	15	2	13	5	6
Egg rolls (3)	1	400	44	6	38	14	19
Extreme Sausage Sandwich	1	670	32	2	30	28	47
Fish & Chips, small	1	630	61	5	56	19	35
French fries, curly – large	1	570	63	7	56	8	32
French fries, curly – regular	1	420	46	5	41	6	24
French fries, curly – small	1	280	30	3	27	4	15
French Toast Sticks	1 svg	430	58	2	56	8	18
Fruit Cup	1	50	14	1	13	1	0
Gourmet Seasoned Croutons	1 svg	100	11	0	11	2	5
Gourmet Seasoned Croutons	1 svg	50	5	2	3	3	3
Hamburger	1	280	29	1	28	14	12
Hamburger Deluxe	1	340	31	2	29	14	18
Hamburger Deluxe w/ cheese	1	430	33	2	31	19	25

	SERVING SIZE	CALORIES	TOTAL CARBS (g)	FIBER (g)	NET CARBS (g)	PROTEIN (g)	FAT (g)
Jack-In-The-Box	...	...	.	.	.	.	.
(cont.)							
Hamburger w/ cheese	1	320	30	1	29	16	15
Hash Browns	5	230	20	2	18	2	16
Hearty Breakfast Burrito	1	780	34	4	30	27	60
Homestyle Ranch Chicken Club	1	720	74	3	71	33	33
Jack's Spicy Chicken	1	550	59	4	55	24	24
Jack's Spicy Chicken w/ cheese	1	630	61	4	57	29	30
Jalapenos, stuffed, 3 pc	1	230	22	2	20	7	13
Jalapenos, stuffed, 7 pc	1	530	51	4	47	15	30
Jumbo Jack	1	580	51	2	49	20	33
Jumbo Jack – bunless	1	230	2	1	1	12	19
Jumbo Jack – no sauce	1	470	47	2	45	20	23
Jumbo Jack w/ cheese	1	670	53	2	51	24	40
Lite Ranch Dressing	1 svg	150	3	0	3	1	15
Low-Fat Balsamic Dressing	1 svg	35	5	0	5	0	2
Meaty Breakfast Burrito	1	630	41	4	37	34	39
Mini Churros (10 piece)	1 svg	650	76	4	72	6	35
Mini Churros (5 piece)	1 svg	320	39	2	37	3	17

	SERVING SIZE	CALORIES	TOTAL CARBS (g)	FIBER (g)	NET CARBS (g)	PROTEIN (g)	FAT (g)
Jack-In-The-Box	...	...	.	.	.	.	.
(cont.)							
Mozzarella Cheese Sticks, 3 pc	1 svg	240	20	1	19	10	14
Mozzarella Cheese Sticks, 6 pc	1 svg	480	39	2	37	20	27
Natural Cut Fries – large	1	620	75	8	67	9	32
Natural Cut Fries – medium	1	460	55	6	49	6	24
Natural Cut Fries – small	1	290	35	4	31	4	15
Onion rings (8 pieces)	1	500	51	3	48	6	30
Pita Snack, Crispy Chicken	1	390	200	39	161	17	170
Pita Snack, Fish	1	380	170	39	131	13	180
Pita Snack, Grilled Chicken	1	310	210	31	179	17	120
Pita Snack, Steak	1	350	200	31	169	19	150
Potato wedges, bacon & cheddar	1 svg	760	53	4	49	21	52
Ranch Dressing	1 svg	310	3	0	3	1	33
Roasted Slivered Almonds	1 svg	110	4	2	2	4	9
Sampler Trio	1 svg	740	450	72	378	26	340
Sausage Croissant	1	580	37	1	36	21	38
Sausage, Egg & Cheese Biscuit	1	590	38	2	36	20	39
Shake, chocolate – large	1	1430	179	2	177	24	69
Shake, chocolate – regular	1	750	95	1	94	12	36
Shake, OREO Cookie – large	1	1450	166	2	164	24	75

	SERVING SIZE	CALORIES	TOTAL CARBS (g)	FIBER (g)	NET CARBS (g)	PROTEIN (g)	FAT (g)
Jack-In-The-Box (cont.)	...	...	.	.	.	.	.
Shake, OREO Cookie – regular	1	760	67	1	66	12	40
Shake, strawberry – large	1	1400	170	1	169	23	68
Shake, strawberry – regular	1	730	90	0	90	11	35
Shake, vanilla – large	1	1290	141	1	140	23	68
Shake, vanilla – regular	1	650	70	0	70	11	35
Side Salad	1	100	11	0	11	2	5
Smoothie, Mango – regular	1	290	72	0	72	2	0
Smoothie, Pomegranate-Berry – regular	1	280	69	0	69	2	0
Smoothie, Strawberry – regular	1	280	69	1	68	2	0
Smoothie, Strawberry Banana – regular	1	290	73	1	72	2	0
Sourdough Grilled Chicken Club	1	530	34	3	31	36	28
Sourdough Grilled Chicken Club – bunless	1	230	5	1	4	30	10
Sourdough Jack	1	680	41	2	39	26	46
Sourdough Steak Melt	1	650	34	3	31	37	40

	SERVING SIZE	CALORIES	TOTAL CARBS (g)	FIBER (g)	NET CARBS (g)	PROTEIN (g)	FAT (g)
Jack-In-The-Box	...	...	.	.	.	.	.
(cont.)							
Southwest Chicken Salad w/ Crispy Chicken	1	310	28	7	21	31	12
Southwest Chicken Salad w/ Grilled Chicken	1	100	11	0	11	2	5
Spicy Corn Sticks	1 svg	220	3	0	3	1	22
Steak & Egg Burrito	1	450	36	1	35	19	25
Supreme Croissant	1	450	36	1	35	19	25
Teriyaki Bowl, Chicken	1	580	106	4	102	26	5
Teriyaki Bowl, Steak	1	650	106	4	102	30	10
Ultimate Breakfast Sandwich	1	570	48	2	46	34	26
Wonton Strips	1 svg	110	13	2	11	2	6
Kentucky Fried Chicken	...	...	.	.	.	.	.
(all salads listed without dressing & croutons)							
BBQ baked beans	1 svg	200	39	9	30	8	2
Biscuit	1	180	23	1	22	4	8
Boneless fiery buffalo wings (1)	1	80	6	1	5	5	4
Boneless HBBQ wings (1)	1	80	7	1	6	5	4
Caesar side salad	1	35	2	1	1	3	2
Chicken little (1)	1	190	20	1	19	6	10
Chicken pot pie	1	690	57	3	54	27	40
Cole slaw	1 svg	180	22	3	19	1	10

	SERVING SIZE	CALORIES	TOTAL CARBS (g)	FIBER (g)	NET CARBS (g)	PROTEIN (g)	FAT (g)
Kentucky Fried Chicken (cont.)	...	...	.	.	.	.	.
Corn on the cob, 3"	1	70	16	2	14	2	Tr
Corn on the cob, 5.5"	1	140	33	4	29	5	1
Country fried steak w/ gravy	1	390	23	2	21	16	26
Creamy ranch dipping sauce	1 svg	140	1	0	1	0	15
Crispy chicken BLT salad	1	340	14	3	11	30	19
Crispy chicken caesar salad	1	320	12	3	9	28	19
Crispy strips (2)	1	250	8	1	7	22	15
Crispy strips (3)	1	380	12	1	11	33	22
Crispy twister w/ crispy strip	1	580	49	3	46	28	30
Crispy twister w/ original recipe strip	1	540	48	4	44	28	26
Double crunch sandwich w/ crispy strip	1	510	36	1	35	27	27
Double crunch sandwich w/ original recipe strip	1	470	35	2	33	27	23
Extra crispy chicken, breast	1	490	17	0	17	38	31
Extra crispy chicken, drumstick	1	150	6	0	6	11	9
Extra crispy chicken, thigh	1	370	12	0	12	18	27

	SERVING SIZE	CALORIES	TOTAL CARBS (g)	FIBER (g)	NET CARBS (g)	PROTEIN (g)	FAT (g)
Kentucky Fried Chicken (cont.)	…	…	.	.	.	.	.
Extra crispy chicken, whole wing	1	150	6	1	5	11	10
Fiery buffalo dipping sauce	1 svg	25	6	0	6	0	0
Fiery buffalo hot wings (1)	1	80	5	1	4	4	5
Fiery buffalo hot wings snack box	1	500	46	4	42	16	27
Fiery buffalo wings (1)	1	80	4	1	3	4	5
Garlic parmesan dipping sauce	1 svg	130	2	0	2	0	13
Green beans	1 svg	25	5	2	3	1	0
Grilled chicken, breast	1	180	0	0	0	35	4
Grilled chicken, drumstick	1	70	0	0	0	10	4
Grilled chicken, thigh	1	140	0	0	0	15	9
Grilled chicken, whole wing	1	80	0	0	0	10	4
HBBQ dipping sauce	1 svg	40	9	0	9	0	0
HBBQ hot wings (1)	1	90	7	0	7	4	5
HBBQ hot wings snack box	1	520	53	4	49	16	27
HBBQ wings (1)	1	80	5	1	4	4	5
Heinz buttermilk ranch dressing	1 oz	160	1	0	1	0	17
Hidden Valley, The Original Ranch, fat-free dressing	1.5 oz	35	8	0	8	1	0

	SERVING SIZE	CALORIES	TOTAL CARBS (g)	FIBER (g)	NET CARBS (g)	PROTEIN (g)	FAT (g)
Kentucky Fried Chicken (cont.)	...	...	.	.	.	.	.
Honey BBQ sandwich	1	310	42	1	41	23	4
Honey mustard dipping sauce	1 svg	120	6	0	6	0	10
Hot & spicy, breast	1	470	15	4	11	38	28
Hot & spicy, drumstick	1	160	5	1	4	12	10
Hot & spicy, thigh	1	380	11	2	9	22	28
Hot & spicy, whole wing	1	160	10	1	9	12	8
Hot wings (1)	1	70	3	0	3	4	5
Hot wings snack box	1	470	41	4	37	16	27
House side salad	1	15	2	1	1	1	0
Jalapeno peppers	1 svg	20	1	1	0	0	Tr
KFC cornbread muffin	1	210	28	1	27	3	9
KFC Creamy parmesan caesar dressing	2 oz	260	4	0	4	2	26
KFC famous bowls-mashed potato w/ gravy	1	700	77	6	71	26	32
KFC famous bowls-rice & gravy	1	790	106	5	101	29	28
KFC Gizzards	1 svg	200	15	1	14	11	11
KFC Kentucky Nuggets (1)	1	45	2	0	2	3	3
KFC Livers	1 svg	180	11	0	11	11	10
KFC mean greens	1 svg	30	4	2	2	3	0
KFC red beans w/ sausage & rice	1 svg	160	26	4	22	24	3

	SERVING SIZE	CALORIES	TOTAL CARBS (g)	FIBER (g)	NET CARBS (g)	PROTEIN (g)	FAT (g)
Kentucky Fried Chicken (cont.)	...	...	.	.	.	.	.
KFC snacker w/ crispy strip	1	300	28	2	26	15	14
KFC snacker w/ crispy strip, buffalo	1	260	30	2	28	15	9
KFC snacker w/ crispy strip, ultimate cheese	1	280	29	2	27	16	11
KFC snacker w/ original recipe strip	1	300	28	2	26	15	14
KFC snacker w/ original recipe strip, buffalo	1	240	29	2	27	15	7
KFC snacker w/ original recipe strip, ultimate cheese	1	260	29	2	27	15	9
KFC snacker, fish	1	320	31	2	29	16	14
KFC snacker, Honey BBQ	1	210	32	2	30	13	3
Macaroni & cheese	1 svg	180	20	2	18	6	9
Macaroni salad	1 svg	180	20	1	19	3	9
Marzetti Light Italian dressing	1 oz	10	2	0	2	0	Tr
Mashed potatoes w/ gravy	1 svg	130	20	2	19	2	5
Mashed potatoes w/o gravy	1 svg	100	16	1	15	2	3
Original recipe chicken BLT salad	1	300	13	4	9	29	15
Original recipe chicken Caesar salad	1	280	11	4	7	28	14

	SERVING SIZE	CALORIES	TOTAL CARBS (g)	FIBER (g)	NET CARBS (g)	PROTEIN (g)	FAT (g)
Kentucky Fried Chicken (cont.)	...	...	.	.	.	.	.
Original recipe chicken, breast	1	370	7	0	7	38	21
Original recipe chicken, breast, w/o skin or breading	1	140	1	0	1	29	2
Original recipe chicken, drumstick	1	110	2	0	2	10	7
Original recipe chicken, thigh	1	260	6	0	6	16	19
Original recipe chicken, whole wing	1	110	3	0	3	9	7
Original recipe filet sandwich	1	480	38	2	36	25	23
Original recipe strips (2)	1	200	7	1	6	21	10
Original recipe strips (3)	1	310	11	2	9	32	15
Parmesan garlic croutons, 1 pouch	1	70	8	1	7	2	3
Popcorn chicken, snack box	1	660	55	5	50	25	38
Popcorn chicken, individual size	1	400	22	3	19	21	26
Potato salad	1 svg	200	24	3	21	2	10
Potato wedges	1 svg	260	33	3	30	4	13
Roasted chicken BLT salad	1	200	7	3	4	30	7
Roasted chicken caesar salad	1	190	5	2	3	29	6
Seasoned rice	1 svg	140	31	1	32	3	Tr

	SERVING SIZE	CALORIES	TOTAL CARBS (g)	FIBER (g)	NET CARBS (g)	PROTEIN (g)	FAT (g)
Kentucky Fried Chicken (cont.)	...	...	.	.	.	.	.
Snack bowl	1	320	34	3	31	12	15
Sweet & sour dipping sauce	1 svg	45	12	0	12	0	0
Sweet kernel corn	1 svg	110	23	2	21	4	Tr
Tender roast sandwich	1	400	29	1	28	34	15
Tender roast twister	1	440	42	2	40	29	18
Three bean salad	1 svg	70	14	3	11	3	0
Toasted wrap w/ crispy strip	1	360	27	2	25	17	20
Toasted wrap w/ original recipe strip	1	340	27	2	25	17	18
Toasted wrap w/ tender roast filet	1	310	24	1	23	22	14
Krispy Kreme Doughnuts	...	...	.	.	.	.	.
Apple fritter	1	380	47	2	45	4	20
Caramel kreme crunch	1	380	49	Tr	49	4	19
Chocolate glazed cruller	1	290	37	Tr	37	2	15
Chocolate iced cake	1	280	36	Tr	36	3	14
Chocolate iced custard filled	1	300	35	Tr	35	3	17
Chocolate iced glazed	1	250	33	Tr	33	3	12
Chocolate iced kreme filled	1	300	35	Tr	35	3	17
Chocolate iced w/ sprinkles	1	270	38	Tr	38	3	12

	SERVING SIZE	CALORIES	TOTAL CARBS (g)	FIBER (g)	NET CARBS (g)	PROTEIN (g)	FAT (g)
Krispy Kreme Doughnuts (cont.)	...	...	.	.	.	.	.
Cinnamon apple filled	1	290	32	Tr	32	3	16
Cinnamon bun	1	260	28	Tr	28	3	16
Cinnamon twist	1	240	23	Tr	23	3	15
Doughnut holes, glazed blueberry	4	220	27	Tr	27	3	12
Doughnut holes, glazed cake	4	210	29	Tr	29	2	10
Doughnut holes, glazed chocolate cake	4	210	29	Tr	29	2	10
Doughnut holes, glazed pumpkin spice	4	210	29	Tr	29	2	10
Doughnut holes, original glazed	4	200	25	Tr	25	2	11
Dulce de leche	1	300	31	Tr	31	3	18
Glazed chocolate cake	1	300	42	2	40	3	15
Glazed cinnamon	1	210	24	Tr	24	2	12
Glazed cruller	1	240	26	Tr	26	2	14
Glazed kreme filled	1	340	39	Tr	39	3	20
Glazed lemon filled	1	290	35	Tr	35	3	16
Glazed pumpkin spice	1	300	42	Tr	42	2	14
Glazed raspberry filled	1	300	36	Tr	36	3	16
Glazed sour cream	1	300	43	Tr	43	2	13
Maple iced glazed	1	240	32	Tr	32	2	12
New York cheesecake	1	340	34	Tr	34	4	20
Original glazed	1	200	22	Tr	22	2	12
Powdered cake	1	290	37	Tr	37	3	14

	SERVING SIZE	CALORIES	TOTAL CARBS (g)	FIBER (g)	NET CARBS (g)	PROTEIN (g)	FAT (g)
Krispy Kreme Doughnuts (cont.)	...	...	.	.	.	.	.
Powdered strawberry filled	1	290	33	Tr	33	3	16
Sugar	1	200	21	Tr	21	2	12
Traditional cake	1	230	25	Tr	25	3	13
Long John Silver's	...	.	.	.	.	.	.
Alaskan flounder	1	250	26	2	24	12	11
Baja fish taco	1	350	29	1	28	9	22
Baked cod	1	120	1	0	1	22	5
Breaded clam strips, snack box	1	320	29	2	27	9	19
Breadstick	1	170	29	1	28	6	4
Broccoli cheese soup, bowl	1	220	8	1	7	5	18
Buttered lobster bites, snack box	1	230	24	2	22	13	9
Chicken plank	1	140	9	0	9	8	8
Chicken sandwich	1	360	40	3	37	14	15
Chocolate cream pie	1 slice	310	24	1	23	5	22
Cocktail sauce	1 oz	25	6	0	6	0	0
Cole slaw	4 oz	200	15	3	12	1	15
Corn cobbette w/ butter oil	1	150	14	3	11	3	10
Corn cobbette w/o butter oil	1	90	14	3	11	3	3
Crumblies	1 oz	170	14	1	13	1	12
Fish sandwich	1	470	48	3	45	18	23
Fish sandwich, ultimate	1	530	49	3	46	21	28
Fish, battered	1	260	17	0	17	12	16
Fries, basket portion	1	310	45	4	41	3	14

	SERVING SIZE	CALORIES	TOTAL CARBS (g)	FIBER (g)	NET CARBS (g)	PROTEIN (g)	FAT (g)
Long John Silver's (cont.)	...	...	.	.	.	.	.
Fries, platter portion	1	230	34	3	31	3	10
Ginger teriyaki sauce	1 pkt	80	18	0	18	1	0
Grilled pacific salmon, 2 filets	1	150	2	0	2	24	5
Grilled tilapia, 1 filet	1	110	1	0	1	22	3
Hushpuppy	1	60	9	1	8	1	3
Ketchup	1 pkt	10	2	0	2	0	0
Lobster stuffed crab cake	1	170	16	1	15	6	9
Louisiana hot sauce	1 tsp	0	0	0	0	0	0
Malt vinegar	0.5 oz	0	0	0	0	0	0
Pecan Pie	1 slice	370	55	2	53	4	15
Pineapple cream pie	1 slice	290	39	1	38	4	13
Popcorn shrimp, snack box	1	270	23	1	22	9	16
Rice	5 oz	180	37	2	35	4	1
Salmon bowl w/ sauce	1	460	65	4	61	30	8
Salmon, Freshside Grille Smart Choice	1	280	27	3	24	27	7
Shrimp bowl w/ sauce	1	380	64	4	60	21	5
Shrimp scampi (8 pieces)	1	110	1	0	1	16	5
Shrimp scampi, Freshside Grille Smart Choice	1	250	27	3	24	19	7

	SERVING SIZE	CALORIES	TOTAL CARBS (g)	FIBER (g)	NET CARBS (g)	PROTEIN (g)	FAT (g)
Long John Silver's (cont.)	...	...	.	.	.	.	.
Shrimp, battered	3 pc	130	8	0	8	5	9
Tartar sauce	1 oz	100	4	0	4	0	9
Tilapia, Freshside Grille Smart Choice	1	250	27	3	24	25	5
Vegetable medley	4 oz	50	8	3	5	1	2
McDonald's	...	...	.	.	.	.	.
Angus Bacon & Cheese	1	790	63	4	59	45	39
Angus Deluxe	1	750	61	4	57	40	39
Angus Mushroom & Swiss	1	770	59	4	55	44	40
Apple Dippers	1 pkg	35	8	0	8	0	0
Bacon, Egg & Cheese Biscuit, large size biscuit	1	480	43	3	40	15	27
Bacon, Egg & Cheese Biscuit, regular size biscuit	1	420	37	2	35	15	23
Bacon, Egg & Cheese McGriddles	1	420	48	2	46	15	18
Baked Hot Apple Pie	1	250	32	4	28	2	13
Barbecue Sauce	1 pkt	50	12	0	12	0	0
Big Breakfast, large size biscuit	1	800	56	4	52	28	52
Big Breakfast, regular size biscuit	1	740	51	3	48	28	48
Big Mac	1	540	45	3	42	25	29
Big N' Tasty	1	460	37	3	34	24	24

	SERVING SIZE	CALORIES	TOTAL CARBS (g)	FIBER (g)	NET CARBS (g)	PROTEIN (g)	FAT (g)
McDonald's (cont.)	...	...	.	.	.	.	.
Big N' Tasty w/ Cheese	1	510	38	3	35	27	28
Biscuit, large size	1	320	39	3	36	5	16
Biscuit, regular size	1	260	33	2	31	5	12
Butter Garlic Croutons	1/2 oz	60	10	1	9	2	2
Cheeseburger	1	300	33	2	31	15	12
Chicken McNuggets, 10 pieces	1 svg	460	27	0	27	24	29
Chicken McNuggets, 6 pieces	1 svg	280	16	0	16	14	17
Chicken McNuggets, 4 pieces	1 svg	190	11	0	11	10	12
Chicken Selects Premium Breast Strips, 3 pieces	1 svg	400	23	0	23	23	24
Chicken Selects Premium Breast Strips, 5 pieces	1 svg	660	39	0	39	38	40
Chipotle BBQ Snack Wrap (crispy)	1	330	35	1	34	14	15
Chipotle BBQ Snack Wrap (grilled)	1	260	28	1	27	18	9
Chocolate Chip Cookie	1	160	21	1	20	2	8
Chocolate Triple Thick Shake, small	12 fl oz	440	76	1	75	10	10
Cinnamon Melts	1 svg	460	66	3	63	6	19

	SERVING SIZE	CALORIES	TOTAL CARBS (g)	FIBER (g)	NET CARBS (g)	PROTEIN (g)	FAT (g)
McDonald's (cont.)	...	...	.	.	.	.	.
Creamy Ranch Sauce	1.5 oz	200	2	0	2	0	22
Deluxe Breakfast, large size biscuit, w/o syrup & margarine	1	1090	111	6	105	36	60
Double Cheeseburger	1	440	34	2	32	25	23
Double Quarter Pounder w/ Cheese	1	380	40	3	37	48	42
Egg McMuffin	1	300	30	2	28	18	12
English muffin	1	160	27	2	25	5	3
Filet-O-Fish	1	380	38	2	36	15	18
French fries, lg	1	500	63	6	57	6	25
French fries, med	1	380	48	5	43	4	19
French fries, sm	1	230	29	3	26	3	11
Fruit 'n Yogurt Parfait	1	160	31	1	30	4	2
Fruit 'n Yogurt Parfait, w/o granola	1	130	25	0	25	4	2
Grape Jam	1/2 oz	35	9	0	9	0	0
Hamburger	1	250	31	2	29	12	9
Hash Brown	2 oz	150	15	2	13	1	9
Honey	1 pkt	50	12	0	12	0	0
Honey Dressing	1 svg	45	12	0	12	0	0
Honey Mustard Snack Wrap (crispy)	1	330	34	1	33	14	16
Honey Mustard Snack Wrap (grilled)	1	260	27	1	26	18	9

	SERVING SIZE	CALORIES	TOTAL CARBS (g)	FIBER (g)	NET CARBS (g)	PROTEIN (g)	FAT (g)
McDonald's (cont.)	...	...	.	.	.	.	.
Hot Caramel Sundae	1	340	60	1	59	7	8
Hot Fudge Sundae	1	330	54	2	52	8	10
Hotcake Syrup	1 pkg	180	45	0	45	0	0
Hotcakes	1 svg	350	60	3	57	8	9
Hotcakes & Sausage	1 svg	520	61	3	58	15	24
Ketchup	1 pkt	15	3	0	3	0	0
Kiddie Cone	1	45	8	0	8	1	1
Low Fat Caramel Dip	1 pkg	70	15	0	15	0	1
McChicken	1	360	40	2	38	14	16
McDonaldland Cookies	1 svg	260	43	1	42	4	8
McDouble	1	390	33	2	31	22	19
McFlurry w/ *M&M's* Candies	12 fl oz	620	96	1	95	14	20
McFlurry w/ *Oreo* Cookies	12 fl oz	550	88	1	87	13	17
McRib	1	500	44	3	41	22	26
McSkillet Burrito w/ Sausage	1	610	44	3	41	27	36
McSkillet Burrito w/ Steak	1	570	44	3	41	32	30
Newman's Own Creamy Caesar Dressing	2 fl oz	190	4	0	4	2	18
Newman's Own Creamy Southwestern Dressing	1.5 fl oz	100	11	0	11	1	6
Newman's Own Low-Fat Balsamic Vinaigrette	1.5 fl oz	40	4	0	4	0	3

	SERVING SIZE	CALORIES	TOTAL CARBS (g)	FIBER (g)	NET CARBS (g)	PROTEIN (g)	FAT (g)
McDonald's (cont.)	. . .	. . .	.	.	.	.	.
Newman's Own Low-Fat Family Recipe Italian Dressing	1.5 fl oz	60	8	0	8	1	3
Newman's Own Ranch Dressing	2 fl oz	170	9	0	9	1	15
Oatmeal Raisin Cookie	1	150	22	1	21	2	6
Peanuts, for sundaes	1 svg	45	2	1	1	2	4
Premium Bacon Ranch Salad	1	140	10	3	7	9	7
Premium Bacon Ranch Salad w/ Crispy Chicken	1	370	20	3	17	29	20
Premium Bacon Ranch Salad w/ Grilled Chicken	1	260	12	3	9	33	9
Premium Caesar Salad	1	90	9	3	6	7	4
Premium Caesar Salad w/ Crispy Chicken	1	330	20	3	17	26	17
Premium Caesar Salad w/ Grilled Chicken	1	220	12	3	9	30	6
Premium Crispy Chicken Classic Sandwich	1	530	59	3	56	28	20
Premium Crispy Chicken Club Sandwich	1	630	60	4	56	35	28
Premium Crispy Chicken Ranch BLT Sandwich	1	580	62	3	59	31	23

	SERVING SIZE	CALORIES	TOTAL CARBS (g)	FIBER (g)	NET CARBS (g)	PROTEIN (g)	FAT (g)
McDonald's (cont.)	...	...	.	.	.	.	.
Premium Grilled Chicken Classic Sandwich	1	420	51	3	48	32	20
Premium Grilled Chicken Club Sandwich	1	530	52	4	48	39	17
Premium Grilled Chicken Ranch BLT Sandwich	1	470	54	3	51	36	12
Premium Southwest Salad	1	140	20	6	14	6	5
Premium Southwest Salad w/ Crispy Chicken	1	430	38	6	32	26	20
Premium Southwest Salad w/ Grilled Chicken	1	320	30	6	24	30	9
Quarter Pounder	1	410	37	2	35	24	19
Quarter Pounder with cheese	1	510	40	3	37	29	26
Ranch Snack Wrap (crispy)	1	340	33	4	29	14	17
Ranch Snack Wrap (grilled)	1	270	26	1	25	18	10
Sausage biscuit w/ egg, large size biscuit	1	570	42	3	39	18	37
Sausage biscuit w/ egg, regular size biscuit	1	510	36	2	34	18	33
Sausage Biscuit, large size biscuit	1	480	39	3	36	11	31

	SERVING SIZE	CALORIES	TOTAL CARBS (g)	FIBER (g)	NET CARBS (g)	PROTEIN (g)	FAT (g)
McDonald's (cont.)	...	...	.	.	.	.	.
Sausage Biscuit, regular size biscuit	1	430	34	2	32	11	27
Sausage Burrito	1	300	26	1	25	12	16
Sausage McGriddles	1	420	44	2	42	11	22
Sausage McMuffin	1	370	29	2	27	14	22
Sausage McMuffin with egg	1	450	30	2	28	21	27
Sausage Patty	1	170	1	0	1	7	15
Sausage, Egg & Cheese McGriddles	1	560	48	2	46	20	32
Scrambled Eggs	2	170	1	0	1	15	11
Side salad	1	20	4	1	3	1	0
Snack Size Fruit & Walnut Salad	1 pkg	210	31	2	29	4	8
Southern Style Chicken Biscuit, large size biscuit	1	470	46	3	43	17	24
Southern Style Chicken Biscuit, regular size biscuit	1	410	41	2	39	17	20
Southern Style Crispy Chicken Sandwich	1	400	39	1	38	24	17
Southwestern Chipotle Barbeque Sauce	1.5 oz	70	18	1	17	0	0
Spicy Buffalo Sauce	1.5 oz	70	1	1	0	0	7
Strawberry Preserves	1/2 oz	35	9	0	9	0	0

	SERVING SIZE	CALORIES	TOTAL CARBS (g)	FIBER (g)	NET CARBS (g)	PROTEIN (g)	FAT (g)
McDonald's (cont.)	...	...	.	.	.	.	.
Strawberry Sundae	1	280	49	1	48	6	6
Strawberry Triple Thick Shake, small	12 fl oz	420	73	0	73	10	10
Sugar Cookie	1	160	21	0	21	2	7
Sweet & Sour Sauce	1 pkt	50	12	0	12	0	0
Tangy Honey Mustard Sauce	1.5 oz	70	13	0	13	1	3
Vanilla Reduced Fat Ice Cream Cone	1	150	24	0	24	4	4
Vanilla Triple Thick Shake, small	12 fl oz	420	72	0	72	9	10
Whipped Margarine	1 pat	40	0	0	0	0	5
Panda Express Chinese Food	...	...	.	.	.	.	.
Beef dishes	...	...	.	.	.	.	.
Beijing beef	1 svg	660	52	4	48	24	41
Broccoli beef	1 svg	150	12	3	9	11	6
Mongolian beef	1 svg	200	16	3	13	15	9
Chicken dishes	...	...	.	.	.	.	.
Black pepper chicken	1 svg	200	11	2	9	14	11
Broccoli chicken	1 svg	180	11	3	8	13	9
Kung Pao chicken	1 svg	300	13	2	11	20	20
Mandarin chicken	1 svg	310	8	0	8	34	16
Mushroom chicken	1 svg	180	10	2	8	14	10
Orange chicken	1 svg	400	42	0	42	15	20
Pineapple chicken	1 svg	230	21	2	19	13	10

	SERVING SIZE	CALORIES	TOTAL CARBS (g)	FIBER (g)	NET CARBS (g)	PROTEIN (g)	FAT (g)
Panda Express	...	...	.	.	.	.	.
Chinese Food (cont.)							
Potato chicken	1 svg	220	18	3	15	11	11
String bean chicken	1 svg	190	13	3	10	12	9
Sweet & sour chicken	1 svg	400	46	1	45	15	17
Chicken breast dishes	...	...	.	.	.	.	.
Pineapple chicken breast	1 svg	230	19	1	18	11	12
String bean chicken breast	1 svg	200	12	2	10	10	12
Thai cashew chicken breast	1 svg	330	17	2	15	15	22
Pork dishes	...	...	.	.	.	.	.
BBQ pork	1 svg	360	13	1	12	34	19
Sweet & sour pork	1 svg	400	36	2	34	13	23
Vegetable dishes	...	...	.	.	.	.	.
Eggplant & Tofu	1 svg	310	19	3	16	7	24
Mixed vegetables, side	1 svg	100	7	3	4	3	6
Mixed vegetables, entrée	1 svg	190	14	5	9	5	13
Rice & noodles	...	...	.	.	.	.	.
Chow mein	1 svg	400	61	8	53	12	12
Fried rice	1 svg	570	85	8	77	16	18
Steamed rice	1 svg	420	93	0	93	8	0
Appetizers	...	...	.	.	.	.	.
Chicken egg roll	1	200	16	2	14	8	12
Chicken potstickers, 3 pc	1	220	23	1	22	7	11
Cream cheese rangoon, 3 pc	1	190	24	2	22	5	8

	SERVING SIZE	CALORIES	TOTAL CARBS (g)	FIBER (g)	NET CARBS (g)	PROTEIN (g)	FAT (g)
Panda Express	...	...	.	.	.	.	.
Chinese Food (cont.)							
Vegetable spring roll, 2 rolls	1	160	22	4	18	4	7
Sauces & cookies	...	...	.	.	.	.	.
Mandarin sauce	1 svg	160	40	0	40	0	0
Potsticker sauce	1 svg	45	10	0	10	1	0
Sweet & sour sauce	1 svg	80	21	0	21	0	0
Fortune cookies (1)	1	30	7	0	7	1	0
Shrimp	...	...	.	.	.	.	.
Crispy shrimp, 6 pcs	1	260	26	1	25	9	13
Kung Pao shrimp	1 svg	230	13	2	11	13	14
Tangy shrimp	1 svg	140	16	1	15	8	5
Soup	...	...	.	.	.	.	.
Egg flower soup	1	90	15	1	14	3	2
Hot & sour soup	1	90	12	1	11	4	4
Panera Bread	*(all sandwiches and salads are full size)*	...	.	.	.	.	.
Asiago cheese bagel	1	330	55	2	53	13	6
Asiago cheese demi	2 oz	160	22	1	21	7	4
Asiago cheese loaf	2 oz	160	22	1	21	7	4
Asiago roast beef sandwich, on asiago cheese bread	1	710	57	3	54	47	32
Asian sesame chicken salad	1	410	31	5	26	32	19

	SERVING SIZE	CALORIES	TOTAL CARBS (g)	FIBER (g)	NET CARBS (g)	PROTEIN (g)	FAT (g)
Panera Bread (cont.)	. . .	. . .	.	.	.	.	.
Bacon Turkey Bravo sandwich, on tomato basil bread	1	840	87	4	83	51	32
Bacon, egg & cheese sandwich	1	510	44	2	42	28	24
Baked potato soup	12 oz	370	33	3	30	8	22
Bear claw	1	460	54	2	52	9	24
Blueberry bagel	1	330	67	2	65	10	2
Broccoli cheddar soup	12 oz	290	24	7	17	12	16
Caesar dressing	1.5 oz	150	2	0	2	1	16
Caesar salad	1	390	25	3	22	12	27
Caramel pecan brownie	1	490	64	2	62	5	25
Carrot walnut muffin	1	430	61	2	59	8	19
Challah bread	2 oz	180	34	1	33	6	3
Cheese pastry	1	400	41	1	40	8	23
Cherry balsamic vinaigrette	1.5 oz	130	7	0	7	0	12
Cherry pastry	1	450	55	2	53	8	22
Chicken bacon dijon panini, on country bread	1	940	96	4	92	59	36
Chicken bacon dijon panini, on french bread	1	780	63	2	61	53	36
Chicken Caesar sandwich, on focaccia	1	860	82	4	78	43	39
Chicken Caesar sandwich, on three cheese bread	1	800	83	4	79	45	33

	SERVING SIZE	CALORIES	TOTAL CARBS (g)	FIBER (g)	NET CARBS (g)	PROTEIN (g)	FAT (g)
Panera Bread (cont.)	...	...	.	.	.	.	.
Chicken salad sandwich, on sesame semolina bread	1	710	101	13	88	31	25
Chicken salad sandwich, on whole grain bread	1	620	77	16	61	31	26
Chipotle chicken sandwich, on artisan french bread	1	1070	87	4	83	54	55
Chipotle chicken sandwich, on french bread		900	53	3	50	49	56
Chocolate chip bagel	1	370	69	2	67	10	6
Chocolate chip muffie	1	270	40	1	39	4	12
Chocolate chipper cookie	1	440	59	2	57	5	23
Chocolate duet w/ walnuts cookie	1	450	55	3	52	6	24
Chocolate pastry	1	340	37	2	35	6	20
Chopped chicken cobb salad	1	490	9	3	6	36	35
Ciabatta	6.25 oz	460	84	3	81	16	5
Cinnamon chip scone	1	530	67	2	65	8	27
Cinnamon crunch bagel	1	430	81	3	78	9	8
Cinnamon raisin loaf	2 oz	180	34	1	33	5	3
Cinnamon roll	1	620	89	3	86	13	24
Cinnamon swirl bagel	1	320	65	3	62	10	3

	SERVING SIZE	CALORIES	TOTAL CARBS (g)	FIBER (g)	NET CARBS (g)	PROTEIN (g)	FAT (g)
Panera Bread (cont.)	...	...	.	.	.	.	.
Classic café salad	1	170	19	4	15	3	11
Cobblestone roll	1	650	123	3	120	12	13
Country loaf	2 oz	140	27	1	26	5	Tr
Country miche	2 oz	140	28	1	27	5	Tr
Cream of chicken & wild rice soup	12 oz	300	29	1	28	7	17
Creamy tomato soup	12 oz	290	28	3	25	4	20
Creamy tomato soup w/ croutons	12.75 oz	370	39	5	34	4	23
Dutch apple & raisin bagel	1	360	77	2	75	8	3
Egg & cheese sandwich	1	380	43	2	41	18	14
Everything bagel	1	300	59	2	57	10	3
Fat-free raspberry dressing	1.5 oz	30	8	0	8	0	0
Fat-free reduced sugar poppyseed dressing	1.5 oz	15	4	1	3	0	0
Focaccia	2 oz	160	29	1	28	5	2
Focaccia w/ asiago cheese	2 oz	160	23	1	22	5	5
Forest mushroom soup	12 oz	250	21	2	19	4	18
Four cheese soufflé	1	480	34	2	32	16	31
French baguette	2 oz	150	30	1	29	5	Tr
French croissant	1	290	31	1	30	6	17
French loaf	2 oz	150	29	1	28	5	2
French miche	2 oz	140	28	1	27	5	Tr
French onion soup w/ cheese & croutons	13.25 oz	250	30	3	27	10	11

	SERVING SIZE	CALORIES	TOTAL CARBS (g)	FIBER (g)	NET CARBS (g)	PROTEIN (g)	FAT (g)
Panera Bread (cont.)	. . .	. . .	.	.	.	.	.
French onion soup w/o cheese & croutons	12 oz	130	20	2	18	3	5
French roll	2.25 oz	180	35	1	34	6	2
French toast bagel	1	350	67	2	65	9	5
Fresh apple pastry	1	380	44	1	43	7	19
Fresh fruit cup, large	1	70	19	1	18	1	0
Fresh fruit cup, small	1	150	37	2	35	2	0
Frontega Chicken panini, on focaccia	1	860	80	4	76	46	39
Frozen caramel drink	16 fl oz	580	83	1	82	6	25
Frozen lemonade	16 fl oz	90	21	0	21	0	0
Frozen mocha drink	16 fl oz	550	78	2	76	7	25
Fuji apple salad	1	410	33	5	28	8	29
Fuji apple salad w/ chicken	1	520	34	6	28	32	30
Gooey butter pastry	1	350	39	1	38	7	19
Greek dressing/ herb vinaigrette	1.5 oz	220	1	0	1	0	24
Greek salad	1	440	15	6	9	10	39
Grilled chicken caesar salad	1	500	26	3	23	35	28
Honey wheat loaf	2 oz	160	30	2	28	5	3
Italian combo sandwich, on ciabatta	1	1040	94	5	89	61	45
Lemon poppyseed mini bundt cake	1	460	63	0	63	6	20

	SERVING SIZE	CALORIES	TOTAL CARBS (g)	FIBER (g)	NET CARBS (g)	PROTEIN (g)	FAT (g)
Panera Bread (cont.)	. . .	. . .	.	.	.	.	.
Light buttermilk ranch	1.5 oz	80	9	1	8	1	4
Low-fat chicken noodle soup	12 oz	140	20	1	19	9	3
Low-fat vegetarian black bean soup	12 oz	170	29	5	24	10	4
Low-fat vegetarian garden vegetable soup	12 oz	120	24	7	17	4	1
Mango smoothie	18 fl oz	330	61	3	58	2	10
Mediterranean veggie sandwich, on tomato basil bread	1	610	102	9	93	22	13
New England clam chowder	12 oz	450	29	3	26	8	34
Nutty chocolate chipper cookie	1	460	54	3	51	5	27
Oatmeal raisin cookie	1	370	57	2	55	5	14
Orange scone	1	460	65	1	64	8	20
Pastry ring, cherry cheese	1	220	27	1	26	3	10
Pecan braid	1	440	46	2	44	8	25
Pecan roll	1	720	88	2	86	11	38
Pineapple upside-down mini bundt cake	1	510	75	3	72	5	22
Plain bagel	1	290	59	2	57	10	2
Plain cream cheese spread	1 oz	100	1	0	1	2	10
Pumpkin muffie	1	250	39	1	38	3	10
Pumpkin muffin	1	530	81	2	79	6	20

	SERVING SIZE	CALORIES	TOTAL CARBS (g)	FIBER (g)	NET CARBS (g)	PROTEIN (g)	FAT (g)
Panera Bread (cont.)	. . .	. . .	.	.	.	.	.
Reduced-fat balsamic vinaigrette	1.5 oz	130	9	0	9	0	10
Reduced-fat hazelnut cream cheese spread	1 oz	80	3	0	3	2	6
Reduced-fat honey walnut cream cheese spread	1 oz	80	4	0	4	2	6
Reduced-fat plain cream cheese spread	1 oz	70	1	0	1	3	6
Reduced-fat raspberry cream cheese spread	1 oz	70	4	1	3	2	5
Reduced-fat sun-dried tomato cream cheese spread	1 oz	70	2	1	1	3	6
Reduced-fat veggie cream cheese spread	1 oz	60	1	1	0	2	5
Reduced-fat wild blueberry muffin	1	360	61	1	60	6	10
Reduced-sugar asian sesame vinaigrette	1.5 oz	90	6	0	6	0	8
Salt bagel	1	290	59	2	57	10	2
Sausage, egg & cheese sandwich	1	550	44	2	42	25	30
Sesame bagel	1	310	59	2	57	10	3
Sesame semolina loaf	2 oz	140	29	1	28	4	Tr
Sesame semolina miche	2 oz	140	30	1	29	5	1

	SERVING SIZE	CALORIES	TOTAL CARBS (g)	FIBER (g)	NET CARBS (g)	PROTEIN (g)	FAT (g)
Panera Bread (cont.)	...	...	.	.	.	.	.
Shortbread	1	350	36	1	35	3	21
Sierra turkey sandwich, on focaccia w/ asiago cheese	1	970	80	4	76	39	54
Smoked ham & swiss sandwich, on rye bread	1	700	55	4	51	40	35
Smoked ham & swiss sandwich, on stone-milled rye bread	1	780	82	7	75	49	29
Smoked turkey breast sandwich, on country bread	1	730	92	7	85	36	23
Smoked turkey breast sandwich, on sourdough bread	1	470	49	3	46	30	17
Smokehouse Turkey panini, on focaccia	1	860	82	4	78	52	36
Smokehouse Turkey panini, on three cheese bread	1	810	83	5	78	54	30
Sourdough baguette	2 oz	160	31	1	30	6	Tr
Sourdough loaf	2 oz	140	28	1	27	5	Tr
Sourdough roll	2.5 oz	200	39	1	38	7	1
Sourdough soup bowl	8 oz	590	117	4	113	22	3
Spinach & artichoke soufflé	1	500	35	2	33	19	32

	SERVING SIZE	CALORIES	TOTAL CARBS (g)	FIBER (g)	NET CARBS (g)	PROTEIN (g)	FAT (g)
Panera Bread (cont.)	. . .	. . .	.	.	.	.	.
Spinach & bacon soufflé	1	570	36	2	34	21	37
Stone-milled rye loaf	2 oz	140	28	2	26	5	Tr
Stone-milled rye miche	2 oz	140	27	2	25	5	Tr
Strawberry granola parfait	1	310	41	4	37	3	12
Strawberry poppyseed salad	1	170	27	5	22	3	6
Strawberry poppyseed salad w/ chicken	1	290	29	5	24	26	9
Strawberry smoothie	18 fl oz	240	51	3	48	5	2
Summer corn chowder	12 oz	260	28	6	22	5	14
Three cheese demi	2 oz	140	26	1	25	6	2
Three cheese loaf	2 oz	140	26	1	25	6	2
Three cheese miche	2 oz	150	27	1	26	6	2
Three seed demi	2 oz	160	27	2	25	6	4
Toffee nut cookie	1	460	59	1	58	5	19
Tomato & mozzarella panini, on ciabatta	1	770	96	6	90	30	29
Tomato & mozzarella salad	1	890	83	6	77	36	47
Tomato basil loaf	2 oz	140	27	1	26	5	Tr
Tuna salad sandwich, on honey wheat bread	1	750	65	6	59	20	47

	SERVING SIZE	CALORIES	TOTAL CARBS (g)	FIBER (g)	NET CARBS (g)	PROTEIN (g)	FAT (g)
Panera Bread (cont.)	...	...	.	.	.	.	.
Turkey artichoke panini, on focaccia	1	750	89	7	82	40	27
Turkey sausage & potato soufflé	1	460	35	2	33	15	28
Very chocolate brownie	1	460	61	2	59	5	22
White balsamic apple vinaigrette	1.5 oz	150	11	0	11	0	12
White whole grain loaf	2 oz	140	27	2	25	5	3
Whole grain bagel	1	370	70	6	64	13	4
Whole grain baguette	2 oz	140	28	3	25	6	1
Whole grain loaf	2 oz	130	26	3	23	6	1
Whole grain miche	2 oz	130	25	3	22	5	1
Wild blueberry muffin	1	390	58	1	57	5	15
Wild blueberry scone	1	390	56	2	54	6	16
Papa John's Pizza	...	...	.	.	.	.	.
Specialty pizzas	...	...	.	.	.	.	.
Cheese Pizza	...	...	.	.	.	.	.
Original Crust – 10"	1 slice	180	25	1	24	7	6
Original Crust – 12"	1 slice	210	27	1	26	9	8
Original Crust – 14"	1 slice	280	38	2	36	12	10
Original Crust – 16"	1 slice	200	41	2	39	12	10
Thin Crust – 14"	1 slice	220	21	1	20	9	12
Pan Crust – 12"	1 slice	410	28	1	27	13	23

	SERVING SIZE	CALORIES	TOTAL CARBS (g)	FIBER (g)	NET CARBS (g)	PROTEIN (g)	FAT (g)
Papa John's Pizza	...	...	.	.	.	.	.
(cont.)							
Pepperoni Pizza	...	...	.	.	.	.	.
Original Crust – 10″	1 slice	210	25	1	24	9	9
Original Crust – 12″	1 slice	220	26	1	25	9	9
Original Crust – 14″	1 slice	310	38	2	36	13	13
Original Crust – 16″	1 slice	330	40	2	38	13	13
Thin Crust – 14″	1 slice	250	21	1	20	10	15
Pan Crust – 12″	1 slice	410	37	1	36	13	24
Sausage Pizza	...	...	.	.	.	.	.
Original Crust – 10″	1 slice	220	25	2	23	8	10
Original Crust – 12″	1 slice	240	26	2	24	9	11
Original Crust – 14″	1 slice	330	37	3	34	13	15
Original Crust – 16″	1 slice	340	40	3	37	13	15
Thin Crust – 14″	1 slice	270	21	2	19	9	16
Pan Crust – 12″	1 slice	420	37	2	35	12	25
The Works	...	...	.	.	.	.	.
Original Crust – 10″	1 slice	220	26	2	24	9	7
Original Crust – 12″	1 slice	230	27	2	25	10	8
Original Crust – 14″	1 slice	330	39	3	36	14	11
Original Crust – 16″	1 slice	350	42	3	39	15	11
Thin Crust – 14″	1 slice	260	22	2	20	11	13

	SERVING SIZE	CALORIES	TOTAL CARBS (g)	FIBER (g)	NET CARBS (g)	PROTEIN (g)	FAT (g)
Papa John's Pizza	...	...	.	.	.	.	.
(cont.)							
Pan Crust – 12″	1 slice	420	338	2	336	14	21
The Meats	...	...	.	.	.	.	.
Original Crust – 10″	1 slice	230	25	1	24	10	11
Original Crust – 12″	1 slice	240	26	1	25	11	11
Original Crust – 14″	1 slice	350	38	2	36	15	16
Original Crust – 16″	1 slice	370	40	2	38	16	17
Thin Crust – 14″	1 slice	280	21	1	20	12	17
Pan Crust – 12″	1 slice	440	37	1	36	15	26
Spicy Italian	...	...	.	.	.	.	.
Original Crust – 10″	1 slice	230	26	2	24	9	7
Original Crust – 12″	1 slice	260	27	2	25	11	8
Original Crust – 14″	1 slice	370	38	4	34	15	11
Original Crust – 16″	1 slice	390	41	4	37	16	12
Thin Crust – 14″	1 slice	310	22	3	19	12	13
Pan Crust – 12″	1 slice	470	38	3	35	15	21
Garden Fresh	...	...	.	.	.	.	.
Original Crust – 10″	1 slice	190	26	2	24	8	6
Original Crust – 12″	1 slice	200	28	2	26	8	7
Original Crust – 14″	1 slice	280	39	2	37	11	9
Original Crust – 16″	1 slice	290	42	3	39	12	9
Thin Crust – 14″	1 slice	210	23	2	21	8	11

	SERVING SIZE	CALORIES	TOTAL CARBS (g)	FIBER (g)	NET CARBS (g)	PROTEIN (g)	FAT (g)
Papa John's Pizza	. . .	. . .	.	.	.	.	.
(cont.)							
Pan Crust – 12″	1 slice	370	39	2	37	11	19
Tuscan Six Cheese							
Original Crust – 10″	1 slice	210	26	1	25	10	8
Original Crust – 12″	1 slice	230	27	1	26	11	9
Original Crust – 14″	1 slice	320	38	2	36	15	13
Original Crust – 16″	1 slice	330	41	2	39	15	13
Thin Crust – 14″	1 slice	250	21	1	20	12	14
Pan Crust – 12″	1 slice	410	37	1	36	15	23
Spinach Alfredo							
Original Crust – 10″	1 slice	190	24	1	23	8	7
Original Crust – 12″	1 slice	210	26	1	25	8	8
Original Crust – 14″	1 slice	280	36	2	34	11	11
Original Crust – 16″	1 slice	310	39	2	37	12	12
Thin Crust – 14″	1 slice	220	19	1	18	8	13
Pan Crust – 12″	1 slice	380	35	1	34	11	22
BBQ Chicken & Bacon							
Original Crust – 10″	1 slice	220	30	1	29	10	8
Original Crust – 12″	1 slice	240	32	1	31	11	8
Original Crust – 14″	1 slice	340	44	2	42	15	11
Original Crust – 16″	1 slice	350	47	2	45	16	12

	SERVING SIZE	CALORIES	TOTAL CARBS (g)	FIBER (g)	NET CARBS (g)	PROTEIN (g)	FAT (g)
Papa John's Pizza	...	...	.	.	.	.	.
(cont.)							
Thin Crust – 14"	1 slice	270	27	Tr	26	12	13
Pan Crust – 12"	1 slice	430	43	1	42	15	22
Hawaiian BBQ Chicken							
Original Crust – 10"	1 slice	230	31	1	30	10	8
Original Crust – 12"	1 slice	240	33	1	32	11	8
Original Crust – 14"	1 slice	340	46	2	44	16	11
Original Crust – 16"	1 slice	360	49	2	47	16	12
Thin Crust – 14"	1 slice	290	31	1	30	13	14
Pan Crust – 12"	1 slice	440	45	1	44	15	22
Sides and Desserts							
Breadsticks	2 sticks	290	53	2	51	9	5
Garlic Parmesan Breadsticks	2 sticks	330	54	2	52	10	10
Cheesesticks	4 sticks	370	42	2	40	15	16
Chickenstrips	2 strips	160	10	0	10	10	8
Wings, Buffalo	2 wings	160	1	1	0	14	11
Wings, BBQ	2 wings	160	4	0	4	14	10
Wings, Honey Chipotle	2 wings	190	8	0	8	12	12
Cinnapie	4 sticks	560	89	3	86	9	19
Apple Pie	4 sticks	480	89	3	86	9	10
Sweetsticks	4 sticks	570	98	3	95	12	15
Chocolate Pastry Delights	1 pastry	180	18	1	17	2	11
Sauces							
Barbecue	1 cup	45	11	0	11	0	0
Buffalo	1 cup	15	2	0	2	0	Tr

	SERVING SIZE	CALORIES	TOTAL CARBS (g)	FIBER (g)	NET CARBS (g)	PROTEIN (g)	FAT (g)
Papa John's Pizza	...	...	.	.	.	.	.
(cont.)							
Ranch	1 cup	100	1	0	1	1	10
Blue Cheese	1 cup	160	1	0	1	1	16
Special Garlic	1 cup	150	0	0	0	0	17
Pizza	1 cup	20	3	0	3	0	1
Cheese	1 cup	40	2	0	2	1	4
Honey Mustard	1 cup	150	5	0	5	0	15
Pizza Hut	...	...	.	.	.	.	.
Appetizers	...	...	.	.	.	.	.
Baked hot wings	2 pc	120	1	0	1	11	7
Baked mild wings	2 pc	110	1	0	1	11	7
Breadsticks, each	1	140	18	1	17	4	6
Cheese breadsticks, each	1 svg	180	20	1	19	7	7
Marinara dipping sauce	3 oz	60	12	2	10	2	0
Stuffed pizza rolls, each	1	230	24	1	23	9	11
Wing blue cheese dipping sauce	1.5 oz	230	2	0	2	1	24
Wing ranch dipping sauce	1.5 oz	220	3	0	3	1	23
Fit 'n delicious pizza (⅛ of 12″ pizza)							
All natural chicken, mushrooms & jalapeno	1 slice	180	22	1	21	12	5
All natural chicken, red onion & green pepper	1 slice	180	24	1	23	11	5

	SERVING SIZE	CALORIES	TOTAL CARBS (g)	FIBER (g)	NET CARBS (g)	PROTEIN (g)	FAT (g)
Pizza Hut (cont.)	...	...	.	.	.	.	.
Diced red tomato, mushroom & jalapeno	1 slice	150	23	2	21	6	4
Green pepper, red onion & diced red tomato	1 slice	150	24	2	22	6	4
Ham, pineapple & diced tomato	1 slice	160	24	1	23	7	5
Ham, red onion & mushroom	1 slice	160	23	1	22	8	5
Hand-tossed style pizza (⅛ of 12″ pizza)	...	...	.	.	.	.	.
All natural Italian sausage & red onion	1 slice	240	26	2	24	10	10
All natural pepperoni	1 slice	230	25	1	24	10	10
All natural pepperoni & mushroom	1 slice	210	26	2	24	9	8
Cheese only	1 slice	220	26	1	25	10	8
Dan's original	1 slice	260	26	2	24	11	12
Ham & pineapple	1 slice	200	27	1	26	9	6
Hawaiian luau	1 slice	230	27	1	26	10	10
Meat lover's	1 slice	310	26	2	24	14	17
Spicy Sicilian	1 slice	250	26	2	24	11	11
Supreme	1 slice	260	26	2	24	11	12
Triple meat Italiano	1 slice	260	25	2	23	12	12
Veggie lover's	1 slice	200	27	2	25	8	7
Pan pizza (⅛ of 12″ pizza)	...	...	.	.	.	.	.

	SERVING SIZE	CALORIES	TOTAL CARBS (g)	FIBER (g)	NET CARBS (g)	PROTEIN (g)	FAT (g)
Pizza Hut (cont.)	. . .	. . .	.	.	.	.	.
All natural Italian sausage & red onion	1 slice	260	28	2	26	11	11
All natural pepperoni	1 slice	250	26	1	25	10	11
All natural pepperoni & mushroom	1 slice	230	27	1	26	10	9
Cheese only	1 slice	230	27	1	26	10	9
Dan's original	1 slice	270	27	2	25	12	13
Ham & pineapple	1 slice	220	28	1	27	9	8
Hawaiian luau	1 slice	260	28	1	27	11	10
Meat lover's	1 slice	330	27	1	26	15	18
Spicy Sicilian	1 slice	270	27	2	25	11	12
Supreme	1 slice	280	27	2	25	12	13
Triple meat Italiano	1 slice	280	27	1	26	12	13
Veggie lover's	1 slice	220	28	2	26	9	8
Stuffed crust pizza (⅛ of 14″ pizza)	. . .	. . .	.	.	.	.	.
All natural Italian sausage & red onion	1 slice	390	40	2	38	17	18
All natural pepperoni	1 slice	380	39	2	37	16	18
All natural pepperoni & mushroom	1 slice	350	39	2	37	15	15
Cheese only	1 slice	340	39	2	37	15	14
Dan's original	1 slice	440	40	2	38	20	22
Ham & pineapple	1 slice	330	41	2	39	15	13
Hawaiian luau	1 slice	360	41	2	39	16	14
Meat lover's	1 slice	480	39	2	37	22	26

	SERVING SIZE	CALORIES	TOTAL CARBS (g)	FIBER (g)	NET CARBS (g)	PROTEIN (g)	FAT (g)
Pizza Hut (cont.)	...	...	·	·	·	·	·
Spicy Sicilian	1 slice	430	40	2	38	19	21
Supreme	1 slice	410	40	3	37	18	20
Triple meat Italiano	1 slice	440	40	2	38	21	23
Veggie lover's	1 slice	330	40	3	37	14	13
Thin & crispy pizza (⅛ of 12″ pizza)	...	...	·	·	·	·	·
All natural Italian sausage & red onion	1 slice	220	23	1	22	9	10
All natural pepperoni	1 slice	200	21	1	20	9	9
All natural pepperoni & mushroom	1 slice	190	22	1	21	8	7
Cheese only	1 slice	190	22	1	21	9	8
Dan's original	1 slice	230	22	1	21	10	11
Ham & pineapple	1 slice	180	23	1	22	8	6
Hawaiian luau	1 slice	220	23	1	22	10	10
Meat lover's	1 slice	290	22	1	21	13	16
Spicy Sicilian	1 slice	230	22	1	21	10	11
Supreme	1 slice	230	23	1	22	10	11
Triple meat Italiano	1 slice	230	22	1	21	11	12
Veggie lover's	1 slice	180	23	1	22	7	6
Popeyes Louisiana Kitchen	...	...	·	·	·	·	·
Biscuits	1 svg	240	26	1	25	4	13
Butterfly shrimp	1 svg	310	22	2	20	13	19
Cajun rice	1 svg	170	22	2	20	8	6
Cajun wing segments	6 pc	600	19	0	19	34	43
Chicken biscuit	1	350	30	Tr	30	13	20

	SERVING SIZE	CALORIES	TOTAL CARBS (g)	FIBER (g)	NET CARBS (g)	PROTEIN (g)	FAT (g)
Popeyes Louisiana Kitchen (cont.)	...	...	.	.	.	.	.
Chicken bowl	1	570	44	8	36	35	29
Chicken étouffée	1 svg	160	6	2	4	12	10
Chicken sausage jambalaya	1 svg	220	20	1	19	10	11
Cinnamon apple turnover	1	250	34	2	32	3	12
Coleslaw	1 svg	260	14	9	5	Tr	23
Corn on the cobb	1	190	37	4	33	6	2
Crawfish étouffée	1 svg	180	25	2	23	7	5
Crispy chicken sandwich	1	560	56	3	53	33	23
Delta Mini	1	300	30	1	29	15	13
French fries	1 svg	310	35	3	32	4	17
Green beans	1 svg	70	14	2	12	2	1
Grilled chicken sandwich	1	360	46	2	44	21	10
Loaded chicken wrap	1	400	44	4	40	19	17
Louisiana Travelers, mild tenders	3 pc	380	24	0	24	33	17
Louisiana Travelers, nuggets	6 pc	220	13	Tr	13	15	12
Louisiana Travelers, spicy tenders	3 pc	410	30	0	30	33	17
Mashed potatoes & gravy	1 svg	120	18	2	16	3	4
Mashed potatoes, no gravy	1 svg	100	17	Tr	17	1	3
Mild chicken, breast	1	350	8	0	8	33	20

	SERVING SIZE	CALORIES	TOTAL CARBS (g)	FIBER (g)	NET CARBS (g)	PROTEIN (g)	FAT (g)
Popeyes Louisiana Kitchen (cont.)	...	...	.	.	.	.	.
Mild chicken, breast, no skin & breading	1	120	0	0	0	24	2
Mild chicken, leg	1	110	3	0	3	11	7
Mild chicken, leg, no skin & breading	1	50	0	0	0	9	2
Mild chicken, strips, no skin & breading	2 pc	130	3	0	3	25	3
Mild chicken, thigh	1	280	7	0	7	16	20
Mild chicken, thigh, no skin & breading	1	80	0	0	0	11	4
Mild chicken, wing	1	150	5	0	5	9	10
Mild chicken, wing, no skin & breading	1	40	0	0	0	7	2
Po Boy sandwich	1	330	36	0	36	8	17
Popcorn shrimp	1 svg	280	22	Tr	22	12	16
Red beans & rice	1 svg	320	31	17	14	10	19
Smothered chicken	1 svg	210	24	1	23	10	8
Spicy chicken, breast	1	360	8	1	7	31	22
Spicy chicken, breast, no skin & breading	1	120	Tr	Tr	Tr	25	2
Spicy chicken, leg	1	100	3	0	3	9	5
Spicy chicken, leg, no skin & breading	1	50	0	0	0	9	2
Spicy chicken, strips, no skin & breading	2 pc	150	5	0	5	23	4

	SERVING SIZE	CALORIES	TOTAL CARBS (g)	FIBER (g)	NET CARBS (g)	PROTEIN (g)	FAT (g)
Popeyes Louisiana Kitchen (cont.)	...	...	.	.	.	.	.
Spicy chicken, thigh	1	300	7	0	7	15	24
Spicy chicken, thigh, no skin & breading	1	80	0	0	0	12	3
Spicy chicken, wing	1	140	5	0	5	8	9
Spicy chicken, wing, no skin & breading	1	40	0	0	0	6	2
Schlotzsky's	(all salads are listed w/ no dressing)	...	.	.	.	.	.
Albuquerque turkey sandwich	1 small	700	57	4	53	34	37
Angus beef & provolone sandwich	1 small	500	55	3	52	27	19
Angus corned beef reuben sandwich	1 small	620	54	4	50	40	27
Angus corned beef sandwich	1 small	390	53	4	49	27	9
Angus pastrami & swiss sandwich	1 small	610	56	4	52	43	24
Angus pastrami reuben sandwich	1 small	620	54	4	50	41	26
Angus roast beef & cheese sandwich	1 small	530	50	2	48	33	22
Asian chicken wrap	1	540	80	5	75	56	12
Baby spinach & feta salad	1	110	6	3	3	8	7
Baby spinach salad pizza	1	450	80	4	76	18	7
Bacon, tomato & portobello pizza	1	620	75	4	71	28	23

	SERVING SIZE	CALORIES	TOTAL CARBS (g)	FIBER (g)	NET CARBS (g)	PROTEIN (g)	FAT (g)
Schlotzsky's (cont.)	...	...	.	.	.	.	.
Barbeque chips	1	220	25	1	24	3	12
BBQ chicken & jalapeno pizza	1	720	99	3	96	69	16
BLT	1 small	370	49	2	47	14	14
Boston clam chowder	1 cup	180	20	0	20	4	11
Broccoli cheese soup	1 cup	170	12	1	11	4	14
Brownie	1	420	54	3	51	5	22
Caesar salad	1	100	10	3	7	6	5
Carrot cake	1	720	80	3	77	7	42
Cheese sandwich, original-style	1 small	560	51	3	48	28	27
Chicken & pesto sandwich	1 small	380	49	3	46	27	9
Chicken breast sandwich	1 small	340	52	3	49	26	4
Chicken salad	1	290	12	3	9	61	15
Chicken tortilla soup	1 cup	140	15	1	14	8	6
Chipotle chicken sandwich	1 small	380	47	3	44	27	10
Chocolate chip cookie	1	160	22	1	21	2	8
Classic swiss & tomato panini	1	620	63	1	62	33	26
Combination special pizza	1	640	76	4	72	27	25
Cracked pepper chips	1	220	25	1	24	3	12
Deluxe sandwich, original-style	1 small	740	55	3	52	43	38
Dijon chicken sandwich	1 small	380	52	5	47	29	7

	SERVING SIZE	CALORIES	TOTAL CARBS (g)	FIBER (g)	NET CARBS (g)	PROTEIN (g)	FAT (g)
Schlotzsky's (cont.)	. . .	. . .	.	.	.	.	.
Double cheese pizza	1	600	74	3	71	27	21
Feta & portobello wrap	1	620	55	4	51	14	39
Fresh tomato & pesto pizza	1	560	73	3	70	25	19
Fresh veggie sandwich	1 small	340	50	4	46	14	10
Fudge chocolate chip cookie	1	160	22	1	21	2	8
Garden salad	1	50	12	4	8	3	1
Greek salad	1	140	13	4	9	7	8
Grilled chicken & guacamole wrap	1	690	60	8	52	63	36
Grilled chicken & pesto pizza	1	680	75	4	71	72	22
Grilled chicken caesar salad	1	220	12	3	9	53	8
Grilled chicken romano panini	1	570	62	1	61	70	16
Ham & cheese sandwich, original-style	1 small	510	54	3	51	31	19
Ham & turkey chef salad	1	250	14	4	10	22	13
Hearty vegetable beef soup	1 cup	60	7	1	6	3	3
Homestyle tuna sandwich	1 small	380	48	3	45	22	11
Homestyle tuna wrap	1	460	55	4	51	23	17
Jalapeno chips	1	220	25	1	24	3	12
Mediterranean pizza	1	560	74	4	70	21	20

	SERVING SIZE	CALORIES	TOTAL CARBS (g)	FIBER (g)	NET CARBS (g)	PROTEIN (g)	FAT (g)
Schlotzsky's (cont.)	. . .	. . .	.	.	.	.	.
Mesquite BBQ baked crisps	1	140	24	2	22	2	4
Mozzarella & portobello panini	1	490	63	2	61	24	15
New York-style cheesecake	1	350	30	1	29	6	23
Oatmeal raisin cookie	1	150	22	1	21	2	6
Old fashioned chicken noodle soup	1 cup	80	12	1	11	6	2
Original baked crisps	1	140	26	2	24	2	3
Original kettle chips	1	190	18	2	16	2	11
Panini italiano	1	740	67	2	65	43	32
Parmesan chicken caesar wrap	1	560	61	5	56	61	21
Pasta salad	1	70	12	1	11	0	3
Pepperoni & double cheese pizza	1	690	74	3	71	31	30
Plain chips	1	220	25	1	24	3	12
Potato salad	1	240	29	3	26	3	13
Potato w/ bacon soup	1 cup	180	22	1	21	4	10
Salt & vinegar chips	1	220	25	1	24	3	12
Santa Fe chicken sandwich	1 small	430	53	3	50	31	10
Side salad	1	25	7	2	5	1	1
Smoked ham crostini panini	1	640	67	2	65	39	23

	SERVING SIZE	CALORIES	TOTAL CARBS (g)	FIBER (g)	NET CARBS (g)	PROTEIN (g)	FAT (g)
Schlotzsky's (cont.)	. . .	. . .	.	.	.	.	.
Smoked turkey & guacamole panini	1	600	69	5	64	32	21
Smoked turkey & jalapeno pizza	1	650	78	4	74	36	21
Smoked turkey breast sandwich	1 small	350	52	2	50	20	6
Smoked turkey reuben sandwich	1 small	610	57	4	53	34	26
Sour cream & onion chips	1	220	25	1	24	3	12
Sugar cookie	1	160	22	0	22	2	7
Texas Schlotzsky's sandwich	1 small	540	51	2	49	32	23
Thai chicken pizza	1	720	85	4	81	71	23
The original sandwich	1 small	560	52	3	49	28	26
Timberline chile	1 cup	280	31	7	24	18	9
Tomato basil soup	1 cup	200	30	2	28	6	5
Turkey & guacamole sandwich	1 small	370	54	4	50	21	7
Turkey bacon club sandwich	1 small	560	51	3	48	32	25
Turkey chef salad	1	310	14	4	10	26	18
Turkey sandwich, original-style	1 small	600	54	3	51	34	27
Vegetarian special pizza	1	540	74	4	70	22	17
Vegetarian vegetable soup	1 cup	100	22	5	17	2	1
White chocolate macadamia nut cookie	1	170	21	1	20	2	9
Wisconsin cheese soup	1 cup	260	20	0	20	4	20

	SERVING SIZE	CALORIES	TOTAL CARBS (g)	FIBER (g)	NET CARBS (g)	PROTEIN (g)	FAT (g)
Sonic	...	...	.	.	.	.	.
Apple slices	1 svg	35	9	2	7	0	0
Apple slices w/ fat-free caramel dipping sauce	1 svg	120	27	2	25	0	0
Bacon cheeseburger toaster sandwich	1	670	52	3	49	29	39
Banana cream pie shake	14 oz	590	98	1	97	7	19
Banana fudge sundae	1	440	70	2	68	4	16
Banana malt	14 oz	490	78	1	77	7	17
Banana shake	14 oz	470	76	1	75	7	16
Banana split	1	420	80	2	78	4	9
Barq's Root Beer float	14 oz	300	56	0	56	3	8
BBQ sauce	1 oz	45	11	0	11	0	0
BLT toaster sandwich	1	500	45	2	43	17	29
Blue coconut Creamslush Treat	14 oz	430	76	0	76	5	13
Blue coconut slush	14 oz	190	52	0	52	0	0
Breakfast burrito, bacon, egg & cheese	1	450	38	1	37	19	27
Breakfast burrito, sausage, egg & cheese	1	480	38	1	37	18	31
Breakfast Toaster, bacon, egg & cheese	1	530	40	2	38	20	32
Breakfast Toaster, sausage, egg & cheese	1	620	40	2	38	20	42

	SERVING SIZE	CALORIES	TOTAL CARBS (g)	FIBER (g)	NET CARBS (g)	PROTEIN (g)	FAT (g)
Sonic (cont.)	...	...	.	.	.	.	.
Bubble gum slush	14 oz	190	52	0	52	0	0
Burrito	1	370	40	6	34	10	18
Burrito deluxe	1	420	43	6	37	13	22
Butterfinger Sonic Blast	14 oz	580	88	0	88	8	22
California cheeseburger	1	690	57	5	52	29	39
Caramel malt	14 oz	550	90	0	90	7	18
Caramel shake	14 oz	530	88	0	88	6	17
Caramel sundae	1	390	64	0	64	4	13
Ched "r" bites	12 pc	280	22	1	21	13	15
Ched "r" bites	4 pc	330	36	2	34	8	17
Cherry Creamslush Treat	14 oz	440	77	0	77	5	13
Cherry slush	14 oz	200	53	0	53	0	0
Chicken club toaster sandwich	1	740	55	4	51	29	46
Chicken strip dinner	4 pc	930	100	7	93	36	43
Chili cheeseburger	1	660	56	5	51	31	35
Chocolate cream pie shake	14 oz	660	114	0	114	7	19
Chocolate malt	14 oz	550	91	0	91	7	17
Chocolate shake	14 oz	540	89	0	89	6	16
Chocolate sundae	1	410	67	0	67	4	13
Coca-Cola float	14 oz	290	54	0	54	3	8
Coconut cream pie shake	14 oz	580	93	0	93	7	20
Corn dog	1	210	23	2	21	6	11
Country fried steak toaster sandwich	1	670	71	4	67	14	37

	SERVING SIZE	CALORIES	TOTAL CARBS (g)	FIBER (g)	NET CARBS (g)	PROTEIN (g)	FAT (g)
Sonic (cont.)	...	...	.	.	.	.	.
Crispy chicken bacon ranch sandwich	1	610	48	4	44	30	34
Crispy chicken sandwich	1	550	46	4	42	22	32
Crispy chicken wrap	1	480	54	3	51	20	21
CroissSonic breakfast sandwich, bacon, egg & cheese	1	510	29	0	29	18	36
CroissSonic breakfast sandwich, sausage, egg & cheese	1	600	29	0	29	19	46
Diet Coke float	14 oz	220	33	0	33	3	8
Diet Dr. Pepper float	14 oz	220	33	0	33	3	8
Dr. Pepper float	14 oz	310	58	0	58	3	8
Ex-long chili cheese coney	1	660	55	4	51	28	39
Ex-long slaw dog	1	670	60	4	56	24	38
French fries w/ cheese, large	1	580	70	5	65	11	28
French fries w/ cheese, medium	1	420	51	4	47	8	21
French fries w/ cheese, small	1	270	32	2	30	5	13
French fries w/ chili & cheese, large	1	690	75	7	68	19	37
French fries w/ chili & cheese, medium	1	490	54	5	49	14	27

	SERVING SIZE	CALORIES	TOTAL CARBS (g)	FIBER (g)	NET CARBS (g)	PROTEIN (g)	FAT (g)
Sonic (cont.)	...	...	.	.	.	.	.
French fries w/ chili & cheese, small	1	300	33	3	30	8	16
French fries, large	1	450	67	5	62	5	18
French fries, medium	1	330	48	4	44	4	13
French fries, small	1	200	30	2	28	2	8
French toast sticks	4 pc	500	49	2	47	7	31
Fritos chili cheese pie, large	1	940	72	6	66	25	64
Fritos chili cheese pie, medium	1	470	36	3	33	13	32
Fritos chili cheese wrap	1	670	66	4	62	21	39
Grape Creamslush Treat	14 oz	430	76	0	76	5	13
Grape slush	14 oz	190	52	0	52	0	0
Green apple slush	14 oz	200	54	0	54	0	0
Green chile cheeseburger	1	630	56	5	51	29	31
Grilled chicken bacon ranch sandwich	1	470	35	3	32	35	22
Grilled chicken salad	1	250	12	3	9	29	10
Grilled chicken sandwich	1	400	32	3	29	28	19
Grilled chicken wrap	1	400	39	2	37	28	14
Hickory burger	1	580	60	5	55	25	26
Hickory cheeseburger	1	640	61	5	56	28	31

	SERVING SIZE	CALORIES	TOTAL CARBS (g)	FIBER (g)	NET CARBS (g)	PROTEIN (g)	FAT (g)
Sonic (cont.)	...	...	.	.	.	.	.
Hidden Valley fat-free Italian dressing	1.5 oz	40	10	0	10	0	0
Hidden Valley honey mustard dressing	1.5 oz	180	10	0	10	1	16
Hidden Valley original light ranch dressing	1.5 oz	110	14	0	14	3	5
Hidden Valley original ranch dressing	1.5 oz	190	2	0	2	1	20
Hidden Valley thousand island dressing	1.5 oz	190	7	0	7	1	19
Honey mustard sauce	1 oz	90	7	0	7	0	7
Hot fudge cake sundae	1	500	73	2	71	5	20
Hot fudge malt	14 oz	580	87	1	86	7	22
Hot fudge shake	14 oz	570	85	1	84	6	21
Hot fudge sundae	1	440	63	1	62	4	18
Jalapeno burger	1	550	53	5	48	25	26
Jalapeno cheeseburger	1	620	54	5	49	28	31
Jr. *Fritos* chili cheese wrap	1	330	34	3	31	12	17
Jr. bacon cheeseburger	1	410	31	3	28	20	23
Jr. breakfast burrito	1	320	25	0	25	12	21
Jr. burger	1	310	30	3	27	15	15
Jr. *Butterfinger* sundae	1	170	26	0	26	2	6
Jr. deluxe burger	1	350	28	3	25	15	20

	SERVING SIZE	CALORIES	TOTAL CARBS (g)	FIBER (g)	NET CARBS (g)	PROTEIN (g)	FAT (g)
Sonic (cont.)	...	...	.	.	.	.	.
Jr. double cheeseburger	1	570	33	3	30	30	35
Jr. *M&M's* sundae	1	180	26	0	26	2	7
Jr. *Oreo* sundae	1	150	22	0	22	2	5
Jr. *Reese's* sundae	1	160	27	0	27	3	5
Jumbo Popcorn Chicken salad	1	420	32	5	27	21	25
Jumbo Popcorn Chicken, large	6 oz	560	41	5	36	27	32
Jumbo Popcorn Chicken, small	4 oz	380	27	3	24	18	22
Lemon Creamslush Treat	14 oz	430	77	0	77	5	13
Lemon real fruit slush	14 oz	200	53	0	53	0	0
Lemon-berry Creamslush Treat	14 oz	460	85	1	84	5	12
Lemon-berry real fruit slush	14 oz	210	55	0	55	0	0
Lime Creamslush Treat	14 oz	430	77	0	77	5	13
Lime real fruit slush	14 oz	200	52	0	52	0	0
M&M's Sonic Blast	14 oz	600	88	1	87	8	24
Mozzarella sticks	1 svg	440	40	2	38	19	22
Nuts add-on for sundaes	3.5 oz	20	1	0	1	1	2
Onion rings, large	1	640	80	4	76	9	31
Onion rings, medium	1	440	55	3	52	6	21
Orange Creamslush Treat	14 oz	430	77	0	77	5	13
Orange slush	14 oz	200	52	0	52	0	0

	SERVING SIZE	CALORIES	TOTAL CARBS (g)	FIBER (g)	NET CARBS (g)	PROTEIN (g)	FAT (g)
Sonic (cont.)	...	...	.	.	.	.	.
Oreo Sonic Blast	14 oz	540	80	1	79	7	21
Peanut butter fudge malt	14 oz	620	83	1	82	9	29
Peanut butter fudge shake	14 oz	610	81	1	80	8	28
Peanut butter fudge sundae	1	470	58	1	57	6	25
Peanut butter malt	14 oz	670	78	0	78	11	36
Peanut butter shake	14 oz	640	75	0	75	10	34
Peanut butter sundae	1	510	53	0	53	8	31
Pickle-O's	1 svg	310	36	2	34	5	16
Pineapple malt	14 oz	510	82	0	82	7	17
Pineapple shake	14 oz	500	80	0	80	6	16
Pineapple sundae	1	370	58	0	58	4	13
Ranch sauce	1 oz	150	1	0	1	0	16
Reese's Peanut Butter Cups Sonic Blast	14 oz	560	89	1	88	9	19
Regular coney	1	390	32	2	30	17	23
Santa Fe grilled chicken salad	1	310	22	6	16	31	12
Sausage biscuit dippers w/ gravy	3 pc	690	57	0	57	16	44
Sonic bacon cheeseburger w/ mayo	1	780	57	5	52	33	48
Sonic burger w/ ketchup	1	560	57	5	52	26	26
Sonic burger w/ mayo	1	650	55	5	50	26	37
Sonic burger w/ mustard	1	560	54	5	49	26	26

	SERVING SIZE	CALORIES	TOTAL CARBS (g)	FIBER (g)	NET CARBS (g)	PROTEIN (g)	FAT (g)
Sonic (cont.)	. . .	. . .	.	.	.	.	.
Sonic cheeseburger w/ ketchup	1	630	59	5	54	29	31
Sonic cheeseburger w/ mayo	1	720	56	5	51	29	42
Sonic cheeseburger w/ mustard	1	620	55	5	50	29	31
Sprite float	14 oz	290	53	0	53	3	8
Sprite Zero float	14 oz	220	33	0	33	3	8
Steak & egg breakfast burrito	1	590	47	5	42	28	34
Strawberry cream pie shake	14 oz	620	106	1	105	7	19
Strawberry Creamslush Treat	14 oz	450	84	1	83	5	12
Strawberry malt	14 oz	520	85	1	84	7	17
Strawberry real fruit slush	14 oz	210	55	0	55	0	0
Strawberry shake	14 oz	510	83	1	82	7	16
Strawberry sundae	1	380	61	1	60	4	13
SuperSonic breakfast burrito	1	570	48	3	45	19	36
SuperSonic cheeseburger w/ ketchup	1	900	60	5	55	46	53
SuperSonic cheeseburger w/ mayo	1	980	58	5	53	46	64
SuperSonic cheeseburger w/ mustard	1	890	57	5	52	46	53
SuperSonic jalapeno cheeseburger	1	890	56	5	51	46	53
Syrup	1 oz	80	21	0	21	0	0

	SERVING SIZE	CALORIES	TOTAL CARBS (g)	FIBER (g)	NET CARBS (g)	PROTEIN (g)	FAT (g)
Sonic (cont.)	...	...	.	.	.	.	.
Tacos	2	340	35	4	31	8	20
Tater tots w/ cheese, large	1	660	55	6	49	10	44
Tater tots w/ cheese, medium	1	420	35	3	32	7	28
Tater tots w/ cheese, small	1	270	22	2	20	5	18
Tater tots w/ chili & cheese, large	1	760	61	7	54	18	53
Tater tots w/ chili & cheese, medium	1	490	38	5	33	13	34
Tater tots w/ chili & cheese, small	1	290	23	3	20	7	21
Tater tots, large	1	530	52	6	46	4	34
Tater tots, medium	1	320	32	3	29	2	21
Tater tots, small	1	200	20	2	18	2	13
Thousand island burger	1	610	56	5	51	26	32
Vanilla cone	1	180	30	0	30	2	6
Vanilla dish	1	240	36	0	36	3	9
Vanilla malt	14 oz	480	72	0	72	7	18
Vanilla shake	14 oz	470	71	0	71	7	17
Watermelon Creamslush Treat	14 oz	440	77	0	77	5	13
Watermelon slush	14 oz	200	53	0	53	0	0
Subway	...	...	.	.	.	.	.
Breakfast flatbread sandwiches	...	...	.	.	.	.	.
Black forest ham & cheese	1	480	46	3	43	27	22
Cheese	1	460	45	3	42	23	21
Double bacon & cheese	1	560	46	3	43	30	28

	SERVING SIZE	CALORIES	TOTAL CARBS (g)	FIBER (g)	NET CARBS (g)	PROTEIN (g)	FAT (g)
Subway (cont.)	...	...	.	.	.	.	.
Mega	1	750	46	3	43	34	48
Sausage & cheese	1	700	46	3	43	30	44
Steak & cheese	1	520	48	3	45	32	23
Western & cheese	1	490	47	3	44	28	22
Breakfast sandwiches, on 6″ bread	...	...	.	.	.	.	.
Black forest ham & cheese	1	450	47	5	42	27	19
Cheese	1	420	46	5	41	22	18
Double bacon & cheese	1	520	47	5	42	29	25
Mega	1	720	47	5	42	33	45
Sausage & cheese	1	670	46	5	41	30	41
Steak & cheese	1	490	48	5	43	31	20
Western & cheese	1	450	48	5	43	27	19
Cookies & desserts	...	...	.	.	.	.	.
Apple pie	1 svg	250	37	1	36	0	10
Apple slices	1 pkg	35	9	2	7	0	0
Chocolate chip cookie	1	220	30	1	29	2	10
Chocolate chunk cookie	1	220	30	Tr	30	2	10
Double chocolate chip	1	210	30	1	29	2	10
M&M cookie	1	210	32	Tr	32	2	10
Oatmeal raisin cookie	1	200	30	1	29	3	8
Peanut butter cookie	1	220	26	1	25	4	12

	SERVING SIZE	CALORIES	TOTAL CARBS (g)	FIBER (g)	NET CARBS (g)	PROTEIN (g)	FAT (g)
Subway (cont.)	...	...	.	.	.	.	.
Sugar cookie	1	220	28	Tr	28	2	12
White chip macadamia nut cookie	1	220	29	Tr	29	2	11
Yogurt, *Dannon* Light & Fit	1	80	16	0	16	5	0
Flatbread sandwiches	...	...	.	.	.	.	.
Black forest ham	1	320	47	3	44	18	7
Oven roasted chicken breast	1	350	48	3	45	24	7
Roast beef	1	340	45	3	42	27	8
Subway club	1	350	47	3	44	26	8
Sweet onion chicken teriyaki	1	410	59	3	56	26	7
Turkey breast	1	310	47	3	44	18	6
Turkey breast & black forest ham	1	330	47	3	44	20	7
Veggie Delite	1	260	44	3	41	9	5
Hashbrowns, 4 pc	1	150	17	2	15	1	9
Pizza, 8"	...	...	.	.	.	.	.
Cheese	1	680	96	4	92	32	22
Cheese & veggie	1	740	100	5	95	36	25
Pepperoni	1	790	96	4	92	38	32
Sausage	1	820	97	4	93	39	34
Salads (w/o dressing)	...	...	.	.	.	.	.
Fat-free Italian dressing	2 oz	35	7	0	7	1	0
Ham	1	110	12	4	8	12	3
Oven roasted chicken breast	1	130	10	4	6	20	3
Ranch dressing	2 oz	290	3	0	3	1	30

	SERVING SIZE	CALORIES	TOTAL CARBS (g)	FIBER (g)	NET CARBS (g)	PROTEIN (g)	FAT (g)
Subway (cont.)	...	...	.	.	.	.	.
Roast beef	1	140	10	4	6	21	4
Subway club	1	140	12	4	8	20	4
Sweet onion chicken teriyaki	1	200	25	4	21	20	3
Turkey breast	1	110	12	4	8	12	2
Turkey breast & ham	1	120	12	4	8	14	3
Veggie Delite	1	50	10	4	6	3	1
Six inch subs	...	...	.	.	.	.	.
Big philly cheesesteak	1	520	53	6	47	39	18
Black forest ham	1	290	47	5	42	18	5
BLT	1	360	45	5	40	17	13
Chicken & bacon ranch	1	570	49	6	43	35	28
Cold cut combo	1	410	48	5	43	21	16
Italian BMT	1	450	48	5	43	22	20
Meatball marinara	1	580	70	9	61	24	23
Oven roasted chicken breast	1	320	49	5	44	23	5
Roast beef	1	310	46	5	41	26	5
Spicy Italian	1	520	47	5	42	22	28
Subway club	1	320	47	5	42	26	5
Subway Melt	1	380	49	5	44	25	11
Sweet onion chicken teriyaki	1	380	60	5	55	26	5
The Feast	1	540	50	5	45	39	22
Tuna	1	530	46	5	41	21	30
Turkey breast	1	280	47	5	42	18	4
Turkey breast & black forest ham	1	300	47	5	42	19	4
Veggie Delite	1	230	45	5	40	8	3

	SERVING SIZE	CALORIES	TOTAL CARBS (g)	FIBER (g)	NET CARBS (g)	PROTEIN (g)	FAT (g)
Taco Bell	. . .	. . .	.	.	.	.	.
Fresco burrito supreme, chicken	1	340	49	6	43	18	8
Fresco burrito supreme, steak	1	330	49	6	43	15	8
Fresco crunchy taco	1	150	13	3	10	7	7
Fresco soft taco, beef	1	180	22	3	19	8	7
Fresco fiesta burrito, chicken	1	340	50	4	46	16	8
Fresco ranchero chicken soft taco	1	170	22	2	20	12	4
Fresco grilled steak soft taco	1	160	21	2	19	9	5
Fresco bean burrito	1	330	55	9	46	11	7
Volcano taco	1	240	14	3	11	8	17
Volcano burrito	1	800	81	8	73	24	42
Taco salad, chicken ranch, fully loaded	1	960	78	8	70	36	57
Taco salad, chipotle steak, fully loaded	1	950	96	8	88	29	59
Taco salad, fiesta	1	820	81	15	66	30	43
Taco salad, fiesta, w/o shell	1	400	41	13	28	24	22
Taco Supreme, crunchy	1	200	15	3	12	9	12
Double Decker taco	1	320	38	7	31	14	13
Double Decker taco supreme	1	350	40	7	33	14	15
Soft taco supreme, beef	1	240	24	3	21	11	11

	SERVING SIZE	CALORIES	TOTAL CARBS (g)	FIBER (g)	NET CARBS (g)	PROTEIN (g)	FAT (g)
Taco Bell (cont.)	. . .	. . .	.	.	.	.	.
Soft taco, ranchero chicken	1	270	21	2	19	14	14
Soft taco, grilled steak	1	250	20	2	18	11	14
Gordita Supreme, beef	1	320	30	4	26	13	16
Gordita Supreme, chicken	1	300	29	3	26	17	13
Gordita Supreme, steak	1	290	29	3	26	14	13
Gordita Baja, beef	1	360	30	5	25	13	21
Gordita Baja, chicken	1	340	29	3	26	17	18
Gordita Baja, steak	1	330	28	3	25	14	18
Gordita Nacho Cheese, beef	1	320	31	4	27	12	16
Gordita Nacho Cheese, chicken	1	300	30	2	28	15	13
Gordita Nacho Cheese, steak	1	290	29	2	27	13	13
Chalupa Supreme, beef	1	370	31	3	28	14	21
Chalupa Supreme, chicken	1	350	30	2	28	17	18
Chalupa Supreme, steak	1	340	29	2	27	15	18
Chalupa Baja, beef	1	410	31	4	27	13	26
Chalupa Baja, chicken	1	390	29	2	27	17	23
Chalupa Baja, steak	1	380	29	2	27	14	23
Chalupa Nacho Cheese, beef	1	370	32	3	29	12	21

	SERVING SIZE	CALORIES	TOTAL CARBS (g)	FIBER (g)	NET CARBS (g)	PROTEIN (g)	FAT (g)
Taco Bell (cont.)	...	...	.	.	.	.	.
Chalupa Nacho Cheese, chicken	1	350	30	2	28	16	18
Chalupa Nacho Cheese, steak	1	340	30	2	28	13	18
Seven-layer Burrito	1	490	67	10	57	17	17
Burrito Supreme, beef	1	410	52	8	44	17	15
Burrito Supreme, chicken	1	390	51	6	45	20	12
Burrito Supreme, steak	1	380	50	6	44	17	12
Fiesta Burrito, beef	1	380	50	5	45	14	14
Fiesta Burrito, chicken	1	360	49	3	46	17	10
Fiesta Burrito, steak	1	350	48	3	45	14	18
Grilled Stuft Burrito, beef	1	690	79	10	69	26	30
Grilled Stuft Burrito, chicken	1	650	76	7	69	33	23
Grilled Stuft Burrito, steak	1	630	75	7	68	28	24
Half pound beef & potato burrito	1	510	66	7	59	14	22
Half pound beef combo burrito	1	450	51	9	42	21	17
Half pound cheesy bean & rice burrito	1	470	60	6	54	12	21
Cheese roll-up	1	200	19	2	17	9	10
Triple layer nachos	1 svg	340	38	6	32	7	18
Cinnamon twists	1	170	26	1	25	1	7
Crunchy taco	1	170	12	3	9	8	10
Soft taco, beef	1	210	21	3	18	10	9

	SERVING SIZE	CALORIES	TOTAL CARBS (g)	FIBER (g)	NET CARBS (g)	PROTEIN (g)	FAT (g)
Taco Bell (cont.)	. . .	. . .	.	.	.	.	.
Cheesy double beef burrito	1	470	54	6	48	18	20
Bean burrito	1	350	54	9	45	13	9
Caramel apple empanada	1	310	39	2	37	3	15
Grilled chicken burrito	1	440	48	3	45	16	20
Grilled chicken soft taco	1	200	19	1	18	12	8
Crunchwrap Supreme	1	540	71	6	65	16	21
Mexican pizza	1	530	46	7	39	20	30
Enchirito, beef	1	360	35	7	28	18	17
Enchirito, chicken	1	340	33	6	27	22	13
Enchirito, steak	1	330	33	6	27	19	14
MexiMelt	1	280	23	4	19	15	14
Taco salad, express	1	600	57	15	42	25	30
Chicken grilled taquitos	1	320	37	2	35	18	11
Steak grilled taquitos	1	310	37	2	35	15	11
Guacamole, side	1	35	2	1	1	0	3
Salsa, side	1	5	1	0	1	0	0
Sour cream, side	1	30	2	0	2	1	2
Chicken quesadilla	1	520	41	4	37	28	27
Steak quesadilla	1	510	41	4	37	25	28
Nachos	1 svg	330	31	2	29	4	21
Nachos Supreme	1 svg	430	41	7	34	13	24
Nachos BellGrande	1 svg	760	77	12	65	19	42
Pintos 'n cheese	1 svg	170	18	7	11	9	6
Mexican rice	1 svg	130	21	1	20	2	4
Cheesy fiesta potatoes	1 svg	270	28	3	25	4	16

	SERVING SIZE	CALORIES	TOTAL CARBS (g)	FIBER (g)	NET CARBS (g)	PROTEIN (g)	FAT (g)
Taco del Mar	. . .	. . .	.	.	.	.	.
Beef baja bowl	1	830	81	10	71	44	35
Beef enchilada	1	1030	115	13	102	55	37
Beef mondito burrito	1	560	71	6	65	28	19
Beef mondo burrito	1	1070	134	12	122	54	36
Beef quesadilla	1	800	66	6	60	49	37
Beef taco salad	1	930	75	12	63	47	49
Beef taco, hard	1	270	17	1	16	17	15
Beef taco, soft	1	280	28	4	24	18	11
Beef, side	1 svg	200	4	1	3	24	11
Black beans	1 svg	140	24	8	16	7	2
Breakfast taco, flour	1	260	18	1	17	13	15
Butter cookie	1	220	31	0	31	2	10
Cheese enchilada	1	820	112	12	100	31	27
Cheese mondito burrito	1	460	69	5	64	16	13
Cheese mondo burrito	1	870	130	10	120	30	24
Cheese quesadilla	1	710	63	4	59	32	35
Cheese, side	1 svg	110	1	0	1	7	9
Chicken baja bowl	1	790	79	9	70	44	31
Chicken enchilada	1	990	113	12	101	55	33
Chicken mondito burrito	1	550	70	6	64	28	17
Chicken mondo burrito	1	1030	131	11	120	54	32
Chicken quesadilla	1	770	64	5	59	49	33
Chicken taco salad	1	900	73	11	62	47	45
Chicken taco, hard	1	260	16	1	15	17	13
Chicken taco, soft	1	260	27	3	24	19	9
Chicken, side	1 svg	170	1	0	1	24	7
Chips & salsa	1	590	78	5	73	8	27
Chocolate chip & nut cookie	1	240	30	2	28	3	13

	SERVING SIZE	CALORIES	TOTAL CARBS (g)	FIBER (g)	NET CARBS (g)	PROTEIN (g)	FAT (g)
Taco del Mar (cont.)	...	...	.	.	.	.	.
Chocolate chip cookie	1	240	34	1	33	2	12
Cod, side	2 pc	120	13	0	13	10	4
Corn tortillas	2	120	24	3	21	3	2
Diced potatoes	1 svg	60	11	1	10	2	1
Egg & cheese burrito	1	490	59	6	53	22	19
Egg & cheese taco, flour	1	200	17	1	16	9	10
Eggs	1 svg	90	1	0	1	7	7
Enchilada sauce	1 svg	35	7	0	7	1	0
Fish baja bowl	1	880	95	9	86	31	41
Fish mondito burrito	1	510	61	7	54	21	21
Fish mondo burrito	1	840	110	12	98	32	30
Fish taco salad	1	1040	89	11	78	34	61
Fish taco, hard	1	270	23	1	22	10	15
Fish taco, soft	1	270	34	3	31	12	11
Flour tortilla, 10″	1	210	33	2	31	7	5
Flour tortilla, 13″	1	350	57	3	54	11	9
Flour tortilla, 6″	1	100	15	0	15	3	3
Green sauce	2 Tbsp	5	1	0	1	0	0
Guacamole	1 svg	40	2	1	1	1	4
Habanero sauce	2 Tbsp	10	1	0	1	0	0
Hash browns	1	110	13	2	11	1	6
Milk chocolate cookie	1	240	31	0	31	3	12
Mondito breakfast burrito	1	640	62	7	55	29	31
Mondo breakfast burrito	1	1190	110	13	97	54	59
Nachos	1	1190	110	12	98	37	65
Oatmeal, raisin & walnut cookie	1	240	35	1	34	3	11
Oreo brownie	1	400	59	1	58	4	17

	SERVING SIZE	CALORIES	TOTAL CARBS (g)	FIBER (g)	NET CARBS (g)	PROTEIN (g)	FAT (g)
Taco del Mar (cont.)	...	...	.	.	.	.	.
Peanut butter cookie	1	240	27	0	27	4	13
Pinto beans, whole	1 svg	90	20	6	14	6	0
Pork baja bowl	1	790	81	9	72	40	33
Pork enchilada	1	990	114	12	102	51	35
Pork mondito burrito	1	550	71	6	65	26	18
Pork mondo burrito	1	920	132	11	121	43	24
Pork quesadilla	1	770	65	5	60	45	35
Pork taco salad	1	900	74	11	63	43	46
Pork taco, hard	1	260	17	1	16	15	14
Pork taco, soft	1	260	28	3	25	16	10
Pork, side	1 svg	170	3	0	3	20	8
Queso	1/4 cup	80	2	0	2	3	6
Red sauce	2 Tbsp	5	1	0	1	0	0
Refried beans	1 svg	160	24	5	19	7	4
Rice	1 svg	230	45	1	44	4	3
Rice & black beans	1 svg	370	69	9	60	12	5
Rice & pinto beans	1 svg	320	66	8	58	10	3
Rice & refried beans	1 svg	390	69	6	63	12	7
Salsa	1 svg	15	4	1	3	1	0
Sausage	1 svg	100	1	0	1	6	8
Sour cream	1 svg	70	2	0	2	1	6
Spinach tortilla, 13"	1	350	56	5	51	10	10
Taco salad shell	1	280	29	1	28	4	16
Taco shell	1	110	14	0	14	2	5
Tomato tortilla, 13"	1	350	56	5	51	10	10
Triple chocolate cookie	1	230	31	1	30	3	12
Vegan mondito	1	430	70	6	64	13	11
Vegan mondo	1	800	133	12	121	24	19
Veggie taco, soft	1	310	49	5	44	11	8

	SERVING SIZE	CALORIES	TOTAL CARBS (g)	FIBER (g)	NET CARBS (g)	PROTEIN (g)	FAT (g)
Taco del Mar (cont.)	...	...	.	.	.	.	.
White chocolate macadamia nut cookie	1	270	30	0	30	3	16
White sauce	2 Tbsp	120	1	0	1	0	13
Whole wheat tortilla, 13"	1	300	54	8	46	12	5
Tim Horton's	...	...	.	.	.	.	.
Angel cream donut	1	310	46	1	45	4	13
Apple fritter	1	300	49	2	47	4	11
Apple fritter Timbit	1	50	9	0	9	1	2
Bacon, egg & cheese sandwich	1	420	34	1	33	16	23
Bagel BLT	1	450	58	3	55	21	14
Banana cream filled Timbit	1	60	9	0	9	1	2
Beef stew	10 oz	240	25	3	22	17	8
BLT	1	450	53	2	51	18	18
Blueberry filled donut	1	230	36	1	35	4	8
Blueberry filled Timbit	1	60	10	0	10	1	2
Blueberry fritter	1	330	55	2	53	6	10
Boston cream donut	1	250	38	1	37	4	9
Café mocha	10 oz	160	25	1	24	1	7
Canadian maple filled donut	1	260	41	1	40	4	9
Caramel chocolate pecan cookie	1	230	32	1	31	3	11
Chicken noodle soup	10 oz	120	18	1	17	5	2
Chicken salad sandwich	1	380	55	3	52	21	9

	SERVING SIZE	CALORIES	TOTAL CARBS (g)	FIBER (g)	NET CARBS (g)	PROTEIN (g)	FAT (g)
Tim Horton's (cont.)	...	...	.	.	.	.	.
Chili	10 oz	300	18	5	13	21	16
Chocolate chunk cookie	1	230	35	1	34	2	9
Chocolate dip donut	1	210	30	1	29	4	9
Chocolate glazed donut	1	260	39	2	37	4	10
Chocolate glazed Timbit	1	70	10	0	10	1	3
Coffee w/ cream & sugar	10 oz	75	9	0	9	1	4
Cream of broccoli soup	10 oz	160	16	1	15	6	9
Creamy field mushroom soup	10 oz	150	28	1	27	3	3
Egg & cheese sandwich	1	370	34	1	33	13	19
Egg salad sandwich	1	390	52	2	50	17	13
English toffee beverage	10 oz	220	40	0	40	3	6
Flavor shot	1 ml	5	1	0	1	0	0
French vanilla beverage	10 oz	240	39	0	39	4	7
Ham & swiss sandwich	1	440	56	3	53	28	12
Hashbrown	1	100	12	1	11	1	5
Hearty potato bacon soup	10 oz	250	23	1	22	6	13
Hearty vegetable soup	10 oz	70	14	3	11	4	0
Honey cruller donut	1	320	37	0	37	1	19
Honey dip donut	1	210	33	1	32	4	8
Honey dip Timbit	1	60	9	0	9	1	2
Hot chocolate	10 oz	240	45	2	43	2	6
Hot smoothee	10 oz	260	39	2	37	5	10

	SERVING SIZE	CALORIES	TOTAL CARBS (g)	FIBER (g)	NET CARBS (g)	PROTEIN (g)	FAT (g)
Tim Horton's (cont.)	...	...	.	.	.	.	.
Iced cappuccino	12 oz	300	41	0	41	0	15
Iced cappuccino, milk	12 oz	180	39	0	39	3	2
Lemon filled Timbit	1	60	9	0	9	1	2
Maple dip donut	1	210	31	1	30	4	8
Minestrone	10 oz	120	24	2	22	3	4
Oatmeal raisin spice cookie	1	220	35	1	34	3	8
Old fashion glazed donut	1	320	35	1	34	3	19
Old fashion plain donut	1	260	20	1	19	3	19
Old fashion plain Timbit	1	70	5	0	5	1	5
Peanut butter cookie	1	280	27	2	25	6	16
Sausage, egg & cheese sandwich	1	540	35	1	34	19	35
Sour cream glazed Timbit	1	90	12	0	12	1	5
Sour cream plain donut	1	270	27	1	26	3	17
Split pea w/ ham soup	10 oz	150	27	5	22	8	3
Strawberry filled donut	1	230	36	1	35	4	8
Strawberry filled Timbit	1	60	10	0	10	1	2
Tea w/ cream & sugar	10 oz	50	10	0	10	1	1
Toasted chicken club sandwich	1	460	70	2	68	30	7
Triple chocolate cookie	1	250	31	2	29	3	13

	SERVING SIZE	CALORIES	TOTAL CARBS (g)	FIBER (g)	NET CARBS (g)	PROTEIN (g)	FAT (g)
Tim Horton's (cont.)	...	...	.	.	.	.	.
Turkey & wild rice soup	10 oz	120	21	1	20	3	2
Turkey bacon club sandwich	1	440	63	2	61	30	8
Vegetable beef barley soup	10 oz	110	21	2	19	4	2
Walnut crunch donut	1	360	35	1	34	4	23
White chocolate macadamia nut cookie	1	240	31	1	30	3	12
White country bun	1	240	49	2	47	9	1
Whole wheat country bun	1	230	46	4	42	10	1
Togo's	(all sandwiches regular size)	...	.	.	.	.	.
Albacore tuna sandwich	1	660	73	4	69	30	28
Asian chicken salad	1	200	17	3	14	21	9
Asian chicken salad wrap w/ asian dressing	1	670	74	8	66	28	32
Asian dressing	2.5 oz	380	10	0	10	0	33
Avocado & cheese sandwich	1	740	73	9	64	25	40
Avocado & cucumber sandwich	1	560	75	9	66	13	25
BBQ beef sandwich, hot	1	670	85	3	82	40	19
BBQ chicken ranch salad	1	230	31	5	26	20	4
BBQ chicken ranch salad wrap w/ buttermilk ranch dressing	1	630	77	8	69	27	26

	SERVING SIZE	CALORIES	TOTAL CARBS (g)	FIBER (g)	NET CARBS (g)	PROTEIN (g)	FAT (g)
Togo's (cont.)	. . .	. . .	.	.	.	.	.
BBQ ranch chicken sandwich	1	750	88	4	84	42	27
Black forest ham & cheese sandwich	1	670	67	4	63	35	31
Blue cheese dressing	2.5 oz	260	3	0	3	2	26
Broccoli cheddar soup	12 oz	350	28	2	26	10	22
Buttermilk ranch dressing	2.5 oz	250	3	0	3	2	26
Caesar dressing	2.5 oz	150	8	0	8	2	12
Capicolla, dry salami & provolone sandwich	1	1080	69	4	65	73	59
Cheese sandwich	1	800	68	4	64	34	45
Chicken Caesar salad	1	210	17	3	14	24	6
Chicken Caesar salad wrap w/ Caesar dressing	1	550	67	8	59	31	20
Chicken salad sandwich	1	650	74	5	69	26	29
Chicken sandwich, hot	1	630	72	4	68	44	20
Chili	12 oz	310	45	10	35	17	6
Chipotle roast beef sandwich	1	990	66	3	63	66	49
Chocolate chunk brownie	1	430	57	3	54	6	22
Classic white bread	1"	50	10	0	10	2	0
Cobb salad	1	330	12	6	6	29	20
Cobb salad wrap w/ blue cheese dressing	1	680	63	11	52	32	36

	SERVING SIZE	CALORIES	TOTAL CARBS (g)	FIBER (g)	NET CARBS (g)	PROTEIN (g)	FAT (g)
Togo's (cont.)	...	...	.	.	.	.	.
Dark chocolate chunk cookie	1	390	51	1	50	4	19
Dutch crunch bread	1"	50	10	0	10	1	0
Egg salad & cheese sandwich	1	750	70	4	66	31	39
Farmer's Market salad	1	160	20	5	15	7	6
Farmer's Market salad wrap w/ balsamic vinaigrette	1	440	72	9	63	12	14
Fat-free serano grape vinaigrette	2.5 oz	90	23	0	23	1	0
French dip sandwich, hot	1	840	67	3	64	67	33
Fresh mushroom & brie soup	12 oz	310	24	2	22	8	21
Garden vegetable soup	12 oz	120	25	4	21	5	1
Honey wheat bread	1"	50	10	Tr	10	2	Tr
Hummus sandwich	1	650	90	9	81	18	27
Italian vinaigrette	2.5 oz	300	4	0	4	0	32
Low-fat balsamic vinaigrette	2.5 oz	90	16	0	16	0	4
Meatball sandwich, hot	1	690	78	5	73	33	27
Moroccan lentil soup	12 oz	190	34	12	22	10	2
Mortadella, salami & provolone sandwich	1	870	71	4	67	58	41
New England clam chowder	12 oz	370	31	1	30	10	24
Oatmeal raisin cookie	1	360	57	3	54	6	13

	SERVING SIZE	CALORIES	TOTAL CARBS (g)	FIBER (g)	NET CARBS (g)	PROTEIN (g)	FAT (g)
Togo's (cont.)	...	...	.	.	.	.	.
Old-fashioned chicken noodle soup	12 oz	170	27	1	26	10	4
Onion herb bread	1″	50	10	0	10	2	0
Pacific cobb sandwich	1	710	68	6	62	34	36
Parmesan bread	1″	60	9	0	9	3	2
Pastrami reuben sandwich	1	990	67	3	64	52	55
Pastrami sandwich, hot	1	750	69	4	65	43	33
Peanut butter chip cookie	1	420	45	2	43	7	23
Roast beef & avocado sandwich	1	720	70	6	64	46	29
Roast beef sandwich, hot	1	730	67	4	63	58	25
Roasted Yukon baked potato soup	12 oz	460	28	2	26	14	31
Salami & cheese sandwich	1	1100	73	4	69	87	53
Santa Fe chicken salad	1	370	33	10	23	27	16
Santa Fe chicken salad wrap w/ spicy pepitas dressing	1	800	75	13	62	34	44
Sicilian chicken sandwich, hot	1	710	73	4	69	41	28
Southwestern chicken & green chile soup	12 oz	400	21	2	19	18	27

	SERVING SIZE	CALORIES	TOTAL CARBS (g)	FIBER (g)	NET CARBS (g)	PROTEIN (g)	FAT (g)
Togo's (cont.)	...	...	.	.	.	.	.
Spicy pepitas dressing	2.5 oz	340	3	0	3	3	35
Spinach tortilla, for wraps	12″	320	53	2	51	7	8
Sun-dried tomato basil tortilla, for wraps	12″	320	54	2	52	7	8
Taco salad	1	600	36	9	27	26	39
Taco salad wrap w/ taco sauce	1	670	90	13	77	24	26
Taco sauce	1 oz	30	7	0	7	0	2
The Italian sandwich	1	860	71	4	67	51	43
Turkey & avocado sandwich	1	640	74	9	65	36	26
Turkey & cheese sandwich	1	670	68	4	64	42	28
Turkey & cranberry sandwich	1	670	95	4	91	34	19
Turkey bacon club sandwich	1	680	68	4	64	35	32
Turkey, ham & cheese sandwich	1	690	68	4	64	42	29
Turkey, ham, salami & cheese sandwich	1	920	71	4	67	70	41
Turkey, roast beef & cheese sandwich	1	770	69	4	65	59	30
Turkey, salami & cheese sandwich	1	900	70	4	66	69	40
Whole wheat tortilla, for wraps	12″	300	52	6	46	8	8

	SERVING SIZE	CALORIES	TOTAL CARBS (g)	FIBER (g)	NET CARBS (g)	PROTEIN (g)	FAT (g)
Wendy's	. . .	. . .	.	.	.	.	.
Ancho Chipotle Ranch dressing	1 svg	90	3	0	3	1	8
Baconator	1	830	35	1	34	56	51
Baked potato, bacon & cheese	1	460	67	7	60	19	13
Baked potato, broccoli & cheese	1	340	70	8	62	10	4
Baked Potato, Plain	1	270	61	7	54	7	0
Baked potato, sour cream & chives	1	320	63	7	56	8	3
Balsamic Vinaigrette	1 svg	90	8	0	8	0	6
Barbecue sauce	1	45	11	0	11	1	0
Bold Buffalo Boneless Wings	1	520	58	2	56	31	18
Caesar Salad, Side	1	70	4	2	2	6	4
Chicken BLT Salad	1	470	23	3	20	35	27
Chicken Caesar Salad	1	180	8	3	5	28	4
Chicken Club sandwich	1	550	48	2	46	34	26
Chicken nuggets (5 pc.)	1	230	11	0	11	12	16
Chicken Nuggets, (10 pc.)	1	470	21	0	21	23	32
Chili, large	1	280	29	7	22	21	9
Chili, small	1	190	19	5	14	14	6
Chunky Blue Cheese dressing	1 svg	230	2	0	2	2	24
Classic Ranch dressing	1 svg	200	3	0	3	1	20
Crispy Chicken Sandwich	1	360	36	2	34	15	18

	SERVING SIZE	CALORIES	TOTAL CARBS (g)	FIBER (g)	NET CARBS (g)	PROTEIN (g)	FAT (g)
Wendy's (cont.)	. . .	. . .	.	.	.	.	.
Crispy Noodles	1 svg	70	10	0	10	1	3
Double Stack	1	360	26	1	25	23	18
Double w/ Everything and cheese	1	700	38	2	36	47	40
Fat-Free French dressing	1 svg	70	17	1	16	0	0
Fish Fillet Sandwich, Premium	1	470	47	1	46	17	24
French Fries, Large	1	540	71	7	64	7	26
French Fries, Medium	1	420	55	5	50	5	20
French Fries, Small	1	330	44	4	40	4	16
Grilled Chicken Go Wrap	1	250	24	1	23	17	10
Heartland Ranch sauce	1	160	1	0	1	0	17
Homestyle Chicken Fillet Sandwich	1	440	47	2	45	25	16
Homestyle Chicken Go Wrap	1	310	30	1	29	15	15
Homestyle Garlic Croutons	1 svg	70	9	0	9	2	3
Honey BBQ Boneless Wings	1	580	75	2	73	32	18
Honey Dijon dressing	1 svg	250	9	0	9	1	24
Honey Mustard sauce	1	130	6	0	6	0	12
Italian Vinaigrette	1 svg	130	8	0	8	0	11
Junior Bacon Cheeseburger	1	310	25	1	24	17	16
Junior cheeseburger	1	270	26	1	25	15	11

	SERVING SIZE	CALORIES	TOTAL CARBS (g)	FIBER (g)	NET CARBS (g)	PROTEIN (g)	FAT (g)
Wendy's (cont.)	. . .	. . .	.	.	.	.	.
Junior cheeseburger deluxe	1	300	28	2	26	15	14
Junior hamburger	1	230	26	1	25	13	8
Light Classic Ranch dressing	1 svg	90	4	0	4	1	8
Light Honey Dijon dressing	1 svg	100	13	1	12	1	5
Mandarin Chicken Salad	1	180	16	2	14	24	2
Mandarin Orange Cup	1	80	19	1	18	1	0
Oriental Sesame dressing	1 svg	170	19	0	19	1	10
Reduced-Fat Acidified Sour Cream	1 svg	45	2	0	2	1	4
Roasted Almonds	1 svg	130	4	2	2	5	11
Seasoned Tortilla Strips	1 svg	110	13	1	12	2	5
Side Salad	1	35	8	2	6	1	0
Single w/ Everything	1	430	38	2	36	25	20
Southwest Taco Salad	1	400	26	7	19	27	22
Spicy Chicken Fillet Sandwich	1	440	49	2	47	26	16
Spicy Chicken Go Wrap	1	320	30	1	29	16	15
Supreme Caesar dressing	1 svg	120	1	0	1	1	13
Sweet & Sour sauce	1	50	12	0	12	0	0
Sweet & Spicy Asian Chicken Boneless Wings	1	550	67	3	64	31	18

	SERVING SIZE	CALORIES	TOTAL CARBS (g)	FIBER (g)	NET CARBS (g)	PROTEIN (g)	FAT (g)
Wendy's (cont.)	. . .	. . .	.	.	.	.	.
Thousand Island dressing	1 svg	290	9	0	9	1	28
Triple w/ Everything and cheese	1	970	39	2	37	69	60
Ultimate Chicken Grill Sandwich	1	320	36	2	34	28	7
Whataburger	. . .	. . .	.	.	.	.	.
Biscuit	1	300	32	1	31	5	17
Biscuit & gravy	1	530	52	1	51	9	36
Biscuit sandwich w/ bacon, egg & cheese	1	500	33	1	32	16	32
Biscuit sandwich w/ egg & cheese	1	450	33	1	32	13	28
Biscuit sandwich w/ sausage, egg & cheese	1	690	33	1	32	26	49
Biscuit w/ bacon	1	350	32	1	31	8	20
Biscuit w/ sausage	1	540	32	1	31	18	37
Breakfast On a Bun w/ bun	1	360	25	1	24	15	21
Breakfast On a Bun w/ sausage	1	550	25	1	24	25	38
Breakfast platter w/ bacon	1	740	53	2	51	24	45
Breakfast platter w/ sausage	1	930	53	2	51	34	62
Chicken strip	1 pc	200	11	0	11	9	12
Chicken strips	2 pc	380	22	0	22	18	24
Chicken strips	3 pc	580	34	0	34	28	37
Chicken strips salad	1	430	33	4	29	19	25
Chicken strips w/ gravy	4 pc	840	53	0	53	37	54

	SERVING SIZE	CALORIES	TOTAL CARBS (g)	FIBER (g)	NET CARBS (g)	PROTEIN (g)	FAT (g)
Whataburger (cont.)	. . .	. . .	.	.	.	.	.
Chocolate chunk cookie	1	230	33	1	32	2	11
Chocolate malt, medium	1	1050	188	3	185	21	25
Chocolate shake, medium	1	1000	171	3	168	22	26
Chop house cheddar burger	1	1170	56	2	54	55	76
Cinnamon roll	1	390	71	3	68	7	9
Egg sandwich	1	310	25	1	24	12	17
French fries, large	1	530	63	5	58	8	27
French fries, medium	1	400	47	4	43	6	20
French fries, small	1	260	31	2	29	4	13
Garden salad	1	50	11	4	7	1	1
Grilled chicken salad	1	220	18	4	14	21	8
Grilled chicken sandwich	1	470	49	3	46	27	19
Honey butter chicken biscuit	1	610	51	1	50	14	38
Hot apple pie	1	230	29	2	27	3	11
Hot lemon pie	1	230	35	1	34	3	12
Junior chop house burger	1	630	28	1	27	30	44
Justaburger	1	290	26	1	25	13	15
Onion rings, large	1	630	55	4	51	8	42
Onion rings, medium	1	420	36	3	33	5	28
Pancakes w/ bacon	1	630	112	5	107	20	12
Pancakes w/ sausage	1	820	112	5	107	30	29
Pancakes, plain	1	580	112	5	107	17	8

	SERVING SIZE	CALORIES	TOTAL CARBS (g)	FIBER (g)	NET CARBS (g)	PROTEIN (g)	FAT (g)
Whataburger (cont.)	. . .	. . .	.	.	.	.	.
Ranch sauce	3 oz	480	4	0	4	1	51
Strawberry malt, medium	1	1040	188	0	188	19	24
Strawberry shake, medium	1	990	171	0	171	20	26
Taquito w/ bacon & egg	1	380	27	3	24	17	21
Taquito w/ bacon, egg & cheese	1	420	27	3	24	19	24
Taquito w/ potato & egg	1	430	37	3	34	15	23
Taquito w/ potato, egg & cheese	1	470	37	3	34	17	27
Taquito w/ sausage & egg	1	410	27	3	24	17	24
Taquito w/ sausage, egg & cheese	1	450	27	3	24	19	28
Texas toast	1 pc	150	20	1	19	3	7
Vanilla malt, medium	1	940	155	0	155	21	27
Vanilla shake, medium	1	890	139	0	139	22	28
Whataburger	1	620	58	2	56	26	30
Whataburger Jr	1	300	28	1	27	13	15
Whataburger w/ bacon & cheese	1	780	59	2	57	36	43
Whataburger, double meat	1	870	58	2	56	43	49
Whataburger, triple meat	1	1120	58	2	56	61	68
Whatacatch dinner	1	1580	161	8	153	29	92
Whatacatch sandwich	1	460	38	2	36	15	29

	SERVING SIZE	CALORIES	TOTAL CARBS (g)	FIBER (g)	NET CARBS (g)	PROTEIN (g)	FAT (g)
Whataburger (cont.)	...	...	.	.	.	.	.
Whatachick'n sandwich	1	550	65	4	61	26	20
White chocolate chunk macadamia nut cookie	1	250	30	0	30	3	14
White peppered gravy, for chicken strips	1 svg	60	8	0	8	0	5
White Castle	...	...	.	.	.	.	.
Sandwiches	...	...	.	.	.	.	.
White Castle	1	140	14	Tr	14	6	7
Cheeseburger	1	170	15	Tr	15	7	9
Jalapeno cheeseburger	1	180	15	Tr	15	8	10
Bacon cheeseburger	1	200	15	Tr	15	10	11
Bacon jalapeno cheeseburger	1	210	15	Tr	15	11	12
Chicken ring sandwich	1	170	19	Tr	19	7	8
Chicken ring sandwich w/ cheese	1	200	19	Tr	19	8	10
Chicken breast sandwich	1	170	21	Tr	21	11	5
Chicken breast sandwich w/ cheese	1	200	21	Tr	21	12	7
Fish sandwich	1	160	19	Tr	19	8	6
Fish sandwich w/ cheese	1	190	19	Tr	19	9	8
Traditional bun w/ cheese	1	100	13	Tr	13	3	4

	SERVING SIZE	CALORIES	TOTAL CARBS (g)	FIBER (g)	NET CARBS (g)	PROTEIN (g)	FAT (g)
White Castle (cont.)	...	...	.	.	.	.	.
Pulled pork BBQ sandwich	1	170	24	1	23	9	5
Surf & turf w/ cheese	1	390	28	1	27	20	22
Surf & turf	1	340	28	1	27	17	18
Double White Castle	1	250	22	1	21	11	13
Double Cheeseburger	1	300	23	1	22	14	17
Double Jalapeno cheeseburger	1	320	23	1	22	15	19
Double Bacon cheeseburger	1	370	23	1	22	19	22
Double fish w/o cheese	1	290	32	1	31	15	11
Double fish w/ cheese	1	310	32	1	31	16	13
Breakfast sandwiches	...	...	.	.	.	.	.
Sausage, egg, & cheese	1	310	12	1	11	15	22
Sausage & cheese	1	230	12	1	11	8	17
Sausage & egg	1	280	12	1	11	13	20
Sausage	1	210	12	1	11	7	15
Bacon, egg, & cheese	1	190	12	1	11	11	10
Bacon & cheese	1	120	12	1	11	5	5
Bacon & egg	1	160	12	1	11	10	8
Bacon	1	90	12	1	11	3	3
Egg & cheese	1	160	12	1	11	10	8
Egg	1	140	12	1	11	8	6
Hamburger, egg, & cheese	1	220	12	1	11	13	13

	SERVING SIZE	CALORIES	TOTAL CARBS (g)	FIBER (g)	NET CARBS (g)	PROTEIN (g)	FAT (g)
White Castle (cont.)	...	...	.	.	.	.	.
Hamburger & cheese	1	150	12	1	11	7	9
Hamburger & egg	1	200	12	1	11	12	11
Sides & sauces	...	...	.	.	.	.	.
French fries, regular	1	400	25	3	22	3	29
Onion chips, regular	1	480	62	2	60	7	23
Onion rings, regular	1	200	28	1	27	2	9
Homestyle onion rings, regular	1	400	49	1	48	4	21
Chicken rings (3)	1	150	8	0	8	8	10
Chicken rings (6)	1	310	17	0	17	15	20
Chicken rings (9)	1	460	25	0	25	23	30
Clam strips, regular	1	250	5	0	5	8	22
Fish nibblers, regular	1	280	24	5	19	19	16
Mozzarella cheese sticks (3)	1	250	22	1	21	10	14
Mozzarella cheese sticks (5)	1	420	37	2	35	17	23
BBQ sauce	1 oz	35	8	0	8	0	Tr
Fat-free honey mustard sauce	1 oz	50	13	0	13	0	0
Marinara sauce	1 oz	15	3	0	3	1	0
Ranch dressing	1 oz	150	1	0	1	0	17
Seafood sauce	1 oz	30	7	0	7	0	0
White Castle zesty zing sauce	1 oz	120	4	0	4	0	11